NURSE TEACHERS AS RESE
A REFLECTIVE APPRO

C000088269

For Bill and Gilly

NURSE TEACHERS AS RESEARCHERS: A REFLECTIVE APPROACH

Edited by

Sally Thomson MA (Ed), BEd (Hons), RGN, RMN, RCNT, Dip
N Ed, Dip N
Assistant Director of Education,
Department of Nursing Policy and Practice,
Royal College of Nursing,
London, UK

Editorial Advisor:

Moya Jolley MA (Ed), BSc (Econ), SRN, Dip Ed, RNT, Dip N(Lond)
Former Lecturer in Sociology and Nursing Development,
Royal College of Nursing Institute,
London, UK

A member of the Hodder Headline Group
LONDON • NEW YORK • SYDNEY • AUCKLAND

First published in Great Britain in 1997 by
Arnold, a member of the Hodder Headline Group
338 Euston Road, London NW1 3BH

British Library Cataloguing in Publication Data
A catalogue record for this book is available from the British Library

Library of Congress Cataloging-in Publication Data
A catalogue record for this book is available from the Library of Congress

ISBN 0 340 66193 3

Composition in 10/12pt Palatino by J&L Composition Ltd, Filey, North Yorkshire
Printed and bound in Great Britain by J W Arrowsmith Ltd, Bristol

Contents

Preface

The idea for this book arose from two sources. Initially I was, and still am, influenced by Stenhouse's (1975) classic notion of the teacher as researcher. He holds that the curriculum should direct a teacher's personal research and development plan, so that an increasing understanding of one's own work improves teaching. Secondly, from my own studies and supervision of others I began to realize that there was a wealth of learning and knowledge to be gained from the product and process of others' work. However, the use of this text is not restricted to nurse educators, although they provide the focus; any would-be researcher would find the contents of it relevant to the practice of research.

This book focuses upon research undertaken by nurse teachers as they implemented and worked with the curriculum in its broadest context. Each chapter is part of a dissertation submitted in part fulfilment of an honours or Masters degree. The chapters include an account of the research undertaken, its findings and a description and discussion of the research process, and also suggestions are made to avoid the pitfalls of the trial and error learning that we engaged in. This gives insight into the practical issues associated with different methods of data collection and overarching research approaches.

Nurse educators now find themselves operating in a research culture, so there is little or no excuse for initiating change based on hunch. Advances in educational practice can only be evaluated and developed if the principles of research are incorporated into our repertoire of normal custom and practice. This will enable us to achieve equality and status in the higher education sector, and for us to transmit research awareness to our students as a way of life.

Despite this, research activity is something that may seem beyond the reach of many nurse educators. This book aims to demonstrate that there is a manageable way of researching that enhances our professional profile and practice, but is manageable upon a small scale.

How to use this book

There are several ways that this book can be read. First, it can be picked up and digested from beginning to end but I doubt that many would want to adopt this approach. Secondly, it can be dipped into and read by chapter as needed, either to focus upon relevant findings or to gain first-hand accounts of approaches and interpretations of methods. Thirdly, the index can be used to direct you through the text, exploring an approach from several perspectives. For example, Dee Burroughs and I both discuss observation. I describe some frustrations and concerns over the role of non-participant observer while Dee offers a rationale for adopting a semi-participant approach. Similarly, Sue Mullaney and Jane Beeby both use phenomenology as a guiding philosophy and approach to research, but the two interpretations of this method sit at either end of a phenomenological continuum. It is up to the reader therefore to decide which best serves their purpose, or to find the answer to the challenges that each chapter poses.

The second chapter in the book summarizes the research approach, and offers some useful suggestions for maximizing upon and surviving each stage. Because of its nature it could also be as usefully read at the beginning, in the middle and at the end of the book. To gain the maximum use out of this, all that is needed is to dip in and select chapters that seem to be relevant or of interest to you, the reader, in your particular work situation; use the index, and consider some of the references we recommend.

Reference

Stenhouse L (1975) *An Introduction to Curriculum Research and Development.* Heinemann, London.

List of contributors

Marion Allison BA (Hons), RGN, Dip N Ed, RNT
Lecturer in Stoma Care Nursing
City University St Bartholomew School of Nursing and Midwifery
London

Gill M Baker BSc, MSc RGN, PGDE, RNT
Senior Lecturer in Life Sciences and Research
School of Pre Qualifying Nursing
Anglia Polytechnic University
Chelmsford

Jayne Beeby MSc, PGDE, BSc, RGN
Senior Lecturer
University of Greenwich
London

Dee Burrows BSc (Hons), RGN, RM, RCNT, RNT, Dip N (Lond)
Senior Lecturer/Research Associate
Faculty of Health Care and Social Studies
University of Luton,
Luton

Alison Goulbourne M. LITT, BSc (Hons) Dip N, RGN
Nurse Lecturer
Department of Health & Nursing
Queen Margaret College
Edinburgh

Moya Jolley MA (Ed), BSc (Econ), SRN, Dip Ed, RNT, Dip N (Lond)
Former Lecturer in Sociology and Nursing Development
Royal College of Nursing Institute
London

Pat Le Rolland BA (Hons), RGN, RCNT, RNT
Principal Lecturer
University of Greenwich
London

Susan Mullaney BA (Hons), RGN, RSCN, Dip N, RNT
Lecture and Programme Director for Child Health
Royal College of Nursing Institute
London

Valerie Anne Smith BA (Hons), SRN, SCM, MTD
Formerly Senior Lecturer
Queen Charlotte's College of Health Care Studies
Thames College
London
Currently living in Paris and undertaking voluntary work

Sally Thomson MA (Ed), BEd (Hons), RGN, RMN, RCNT, Dip N Ed, Dip N
Assistant Director of Education
Department of Nursing Policy and Practice
Royal College of Nursing
London

1

Reflections

Moya Jolley

Introduction

'And now', as they say in television chat shows, 'for something a little different'. It has been my privilege to be able to watch the creation of this book, over an 18 month period, which has been filled with much activity, and a lot of hard work for all those concerned. The overall aim in compilation has been to provide flexible, free-flowing accounts that take a journey around the subject of 'the teacher as researcher', while also providing informative and stimulating narratives relating to the contributors' own experiences in the field of nursing research.

The past decade has constituted a period of intense upheaval, challenge and difficulty within the field of nurse education. Since the launch of Project 2000 in 1986 and with it the move towards an all-graduate teaching profession within nursing, change has become the order of the day. Old traditions, professional 'sacred cows', entrenched attitudes and values have all, in turn, come under the spotlight of reform. While not seeking to minimize the disruptions reforms inevitably bring, there can be little doubt that standards in nursing are rising and that there is now, more than ever, the need for nurse practitioners to be critical thinkers with analytical skills. One contributor reminds us, quoting Nickersen (1987), that the old attitude enshrined in the phrase 'you are not here to think, nurse' can result in 'blindly following authority, acting without thought for the consequences of our actions, having opinions moulded and our behaviour shaped by illogical arguments, believing the future will be what it will be and taking no steps to make it what it could be'. Modern nursing education seeks to eliminate this unwanted legacy from another era.

Subjects which in the past were not deemed relevant, or were looked upon with suspicious reservation, have now 'come in from the cold' and found a place in the curriculum. Included among these is nursing research, once viewed as a minority sport only for those more mathematically gifted and of a particularly enquiring mind, i.e. those not always prepared to accept what they found in nursing practice simply because 'it had always been done that way'. The encouragement of research mindedness is now seen for what it is, an absolutely essential element in the educational preparation of the modern nurse.

In relation to this aspect one contributor looks in depth at fostering critical thinking within nurse education, defining such thinking as 'a process which involves careful, persistent and objective analysis of knowledge, beliefs or situations in order to judge their ability or worth'. Such skills are needed for students to make their professional contribution to nursing development as a science. The writer also discusses the importance of providing opportunities to develop reflective scepticism and to accept and tolerate ambiguity in nursing situations where no 'right' answer is immediately apparent.

This book consists of a series of research studies carried out by nurses in mid career who have been taking higher nursing education courses which included a research component. The contributions, therefore, are not those of high profile researchers but of highly motivated enthusiastic individuals learning their craft. Because of this, their accounts have a special relevance for those readers starting out on research projects themselves.

Designed not only to be informative and stimulating, which they most certainly are, these accounts provide both warnings and encouragement to those who may choose to follow along the same paths. Among the many aspects addressed are the problems of researcher fallibility, ethical dilemmas, personal learning difficulties and their resolution, problems of confidentiality, choice of research method and data analysis and power relationships and the perceptions of those being researched.

Thankfully, this book does not attempt to adhere to a rigid textural construction but explores freely and thoughtfully wide vistas of the subject, embracing as it does so varying contextual problems, teaching and research conundrums and inevitably raising more questions than it answers in the process! As one contributor remarked 'in attempting to answer questions new questions emerged to tease!'.

The editor of this book has wielded her blue pencil with great sensitivity allowing each chapter to assume its own character and deliver its own message. The result is a collection of highly individual accounts each demonstrating considerable variation in style, format and approach, yet providing a richness in terms of information imparted, problems addressed and experiences shared. This represents a move away from the somewhat predictable textual progression evident in so many research books. Because of the variation in approach an editorial link statement introduces each chapter, thus maintaining the overall thematic connections. The contributors confront and explore a wide range of research problems covering most of those likely to be encountered by novice researchers. The high level of personal commitment and sheer 'stickability' of the researchers themselves comes through clearly in all these accounts.

Honest, often humorous, highly informative and obviously written from a position of 'wisdom after the event', each chapter has much to offer in terms of research know-how, problem solving and how to cope when things threaten to get out of hand! As one contributor wryly observed, her research project constituted 'one of the greatest leaps in learning I have ever experienced'.

The research process in all its stages is addressed throughout the book, but in widely varying contexts, thus providing a range of differing perspectives in each case. The studies encompass both quantitative and qualitative research with interesting insights given into phenomenological approaches, action research and the complexities of triangulation among other things.

All the contributors write with refreshing frankness regarding the challenges confronted in the course of their research and the remedies sought to overcome them: very useful reading for any 'rookie' researcher! For example, concerning data collection one contributor writes 'I had hit a morass of impenetrable, unintelligible information that was insurmountable'. She goes on to share with the reader how she endeavoured to cope with this problem. The writers of Chapters 3 and 4 deal with the personal feelings engendered as a researcher and both authors are sharply self-critical in evaluating their work. Statistical analysis can also be 'a way of sorrows' for those of us less mathematically gifted. The authors of several chapters address this area of difficulty and suggest possible solutions. These and many other problems are not only identified in this book but solutions searched for and problem-solving techniques adopted. Here, learning by doing is sometimes demonstrated; while not always the most favoured learning method, it certainly possesses a lasting durability for the individual concerned. How many of us can still remember vividly such learning experiences from student days!

All the contributors have been generous as well as frank in offering advice arising from their own experiences and also in recommending methods they have found helpful.

It is not a matter for debate that research is an academic discipline both in its theoretical and its factual/experiential aspects which encourages independent thinking and innovative approaches in the nursing context. It also sometimes reveals, as one contributor points out 'how much further there is to go, and the problem then becomes when to stop'.

This book presents the reader with a series of fascinating research studies which should certainly stimulate new thinking and possibly encourage others to 'have a go'. The extensive reference lists should also serve as rich sources of information on all the research addressed here.

Were I embarking once again, as 30 years ago, on a teaching career within nursing, I would find a book such as this both helpful and challenging.

2

Using the research process
Gill Baker

This chapter is essential reading for anyone getting ready to embark upon a research project of any size. It is one that I think you will go back to over and over again at various stages of your work:

- *The stages of the research process identified in Figure 2.1 provide clear milestones and stages for any style of project, large or small, qualitative or quantitative. In qualitative work the boundaries between some of the stages may be blurred, but, nevertheless, they provide a clear map. At least if you discount a stage you will do so with insight.*
- *Much of what is sketched in this chapter is developed in the others. However, the section on choosing a topic is particularly useful.*
- *Gill's use of her own experience will prevent you from falling into similar traps and allow you to foster positive techniques. Finally, it will help you think about publishing your findings which is implicit from the style of this book and explicit in the conclusion of this chapter.*

Introduction

As a nurse I have participated in and planned several pieces of research, in so doing I have gained experience the hard way, i.e. by making my own mistakes. Whilst I am in favour of learning by doing, I do not feel that this means that every nurse researcher has to make the same errors in order to become a competent researcher. Learning from other people's mistakes and benefiting from their experiences as well as from your own seems far more sensible. The ideal way to do this is to carry out research with an experienced researcher until you are confident enough in your own skills and limitations to 'go it alone'. This is not always possible and many nurses may undertake their first piece of research on their own. In writing this chapter I have tried to include all the advice and guidance that has been given to me, together with the suggestions from my own experience that my research students have found useful in the past. This approach means that the majority of the information contained within this chapter has not previously been published, and has been gained experimentally.

> It is difficult to tell anyone how to do research. Perhaps the best thing to do is to make sure that the beginner has a grasp of principles and possibilities; in addition, approaches and tactics can be suggested. (Kerlinger, 1986, cited in Herbert, 1990)

This chapter was written as an attempt to comply with Kerlinger's suggestions and I hope that by reading the advice and suggestions contained within it you will gain some of the benefits of having another researcher available to share her experiences and tips with you.

The research process

> Whatever the scale of the research project, it is suggested that worthwhile research is characterised by a logical approach to solving a problem or obtaining and analysing information. This logical approach is called the research process. (Reid and Boore, 1987)

The research process is a framework of steps that need to be carried out in order for a piece of research to be completed. This framework is often thought only to apply to research using a quantitative approach (e.g. Burns and Grove, 1993). However, the usefulness of the research process lies in the fact that it is a framework that can have its constituent steps rearranged or repeated to suit the type of research being planned. This flexibility means that it is possible to use a research process framework in most research situations.

Following discussion with other nurse researchers and teachers of research skills I identified 15 separate stages in the research process (see Figure 2.1). Some of these stages may occur simultaneously; e.g. it is often sensible to apply for funding at the same time as applying for ethical approval. Other stages are obviously linked together and, regardless of the methodology used, are always performed in a certain order; e.g. data cannot be analysed before it has been collected. As previously stated, stages may be repeated where necessary; e.g. if instruments are substantially altered after a pilot study a second pilot study may be performed to test the new instruments.

The research process is a cyclical process in which, while sharing the findings with others, as part of the writing the research report the researcher will identify further topics that could be researched to extend or aid application of the present piece of research. The stage identified as carrying out a literature search, which is very important at the beginning of most types of research (see Research process framework), should continue

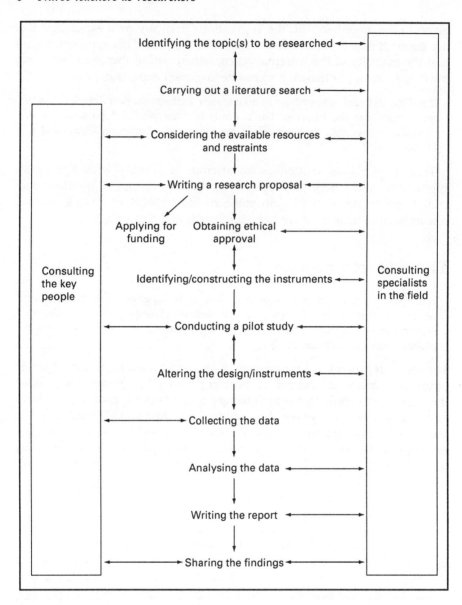

Figure 2.1   Research process framework

throughout the entire research process so that the latest information is incorporated into the study and research report. These aspects of the research process are not fully reflected in the research process framework that I have designed; trying to incorporate these aspects of the process made the framework too confusing to be of any practical help to those wishing to use it to help them in designing their own research studies.

All research has potential ethical dilemmas, therefore it is important to consider ethical issues at every stage of your research. Herbert (1990) lists four questions that researchers should be asking about their research:

- Is your client ('subject') making an informed and free choice in participating in your study?
- Does he or she appreciate all the implications?
- Are your methods ethical?
- Will the individual results be kept confidential?

These are just a few of the ethical areas that an ethics committee (see Obtaining ethical approval) will expect you to have considered in your application. Other important issues to consider are:

- Does your study expose subjects to any physical or mental stress?
- Are you withholding any benefits from the subjects in the control group?
- Are you withholding from the subjects the true nature of your research?
- Are you violating the privacy of your subjects?
- Are there any circumstances under which you would withdraw a subject from the study or use information from the study other than as study data?

For more information on the ethical implications of various research methodologies consult Chapter 3 in this book.

The remainder of this chapter discusses each of the identified stages of the research process in detail. Within each of these sections I have included appropriate advice and suggestions that may make the process easier for both novice and experienced nurse researchers. I have also illustrated this advice by explaining how I completed each stage of the research process whilst undertaking a major piece of clinical research in part fulfilment for an MSc in Nursing from the University of London.

Identifying the topic(s) to be researched

For many nurses wishing to undertake research this can be one of the hardest stages of the research process, for others it is the easiest. The biggest barrier to identifying a topic to be researched may be to be told that you have to carry out a piece of research now! Nothing more effectively clears the brain of any ideas than to be asked to produce an idea with only a few days' notice. If you are undertaking a course in which you have to write a research proposal or undertake the research process, don't leave thinking about the topic to be researched until deadlines are imminent; start thinking of topics that interest you well in advance. If you don't select a research area that really interests you it will be far more of a struggle to keep up the momentum needed to conduct a research project that lasts more than a few days, particularly if you are working largely on your own.

The initial idea for your research can come from: reading literature to keep yourself aware of current issues; carrying out a literature search on a topic that you are already interested in; a meeting with educational, managerial or clinical colleagues; or your current clinical practice. Clinical practice is probably one of the best sources of research ideas for a nurse wishing to undertake his/her first piece of research.

Proposed changes in clinical practice or ward management could/should be examined so that the effects upon staff and patients can be explored, and the implications of the changes can be monitored. Any incident that occurs at work may cause a nurse to examine his/her clinical practice, attitude or beliefs, or those of others. Such examination may identify a research topic.

One other source of ideas for nursing research is that a nurse may be asked by his/her manager to conduct research into an issue that is felt to be important for a particular clinical area. There are a number of potential problem areas that you should explore before agreeing to conduct research to meet somebody else's needs: will you be allowed the freedom to conduct the research as you wish?; will you be allowed to keep all of your original data confidential or will the manager wish to see this in addition to your findings and conclusions?; will you experience any reluctance by colleagues to participate in research that they see as being a management tool? (this is a potential problem that may be particularly important if you are asked to extend another research study to incorporate issues that your manager wishes to have researched); will you be set a completion date that makes it impossible for you to collect sufficient data for your results to be meaningful or a starting date that means that you have not fully thought through the research design before you have to start data collection? These potential problems can also apply to research that is conducted on behalf of a manufacturer or funded by a research grant.

In order to complete my MSc in Nursing I had to submit a research proposal to the University, and then carry out a major piece of research. Since I was also working as a dialysis nurse I decided that it would be easiest for me to conduct my research within this clinical area. Conducting research where you work has a number of advantages and disadvantages e.g. how will objectivity be maintained?; will subjects feel under pressure to participate, or to give you the responses that they feel you want?; how will lack of cooperation affect your professional relationships? Looking back I did not sufficiently consider the potential problems of conducting research where I was working as a nurse, but in this case the support and help provided by my employers did indeed outweigh any of the disadvantages of using colleagues and my own patients as research subjects.

For many years I had been interested in and active in providing patient education, therefore I decided to carry out a literature search into patient education, focused upon education for patients with renal failure who were receiving haemodialysis.

At about the same time the management of the renal unit were expressing concern at the *ad hoc* way in which patients were educated about their treatment regimen. Education took place whenever individual nurses decided that they had time to spare from their other duties or when patients asked for specific information. Thus patients were not being educated in a systematic way geared towards their individual requirements and capabilities. The unit's philosophy of promoting self-care was difficult to implement for many of the patients, since they did not appear to have the knowledge and skills to reach their self-care potential. I was asked to join the education team to design a new educational programme that would promote self-care. Therefore, I decided that part of my research should include measurement of patients' current level of knowledge about their treatment regimen.

After I had received ethical approval for my study (see Obtaining ethical approval) and conducted a pilot study (see Conducting a pilot study) I gained a new research supervisor from the University. When we discussed my research it was decided that the concept of compliance was also important for these patients, and that this topic should be added to the research project.

Reading literature relating to the previously mentioned topics identified two further related topics relevant to my research: the Health Belief Model (Janz and Becker, 1984), and perceptions of the importance of patients receiving information concerning different aspects of their treatment regimen (Goddard and Powers, 1982).

Thus from a combination of discussion with colleagues and supervisors, a review of my clinical interests and responsibilities, and a review of the available literature, I chose my research area as education for patients being treated by haemodialysis, and identified six topics to be included in the study: patient education; current level of patient knowledge with regard to their treatment regimen; self-care; compliance; the Health Belief Model; and perception of the importance of patients receiving information concerning different aspects of their treatment regimen.

Carrying out a literature search (literature review)

All empirical research should be based upon a critical evaluation of the current level of available knowledge. It would be ridiculous to expect everyone who is embarking upon a piece of research already to have an in depth knowledge of every topic that is connected with their research idea; therefore one of the first research activities that will be essential to most researchers is to conduct a literature search.

A literature search involves locating, critically evaluating and summarizing existing information on a problem. Thus the literature search enables you to

> clarify which problems have been investigated, which require further investigation or replication, and which have not been investigated. In addition the literature review directs the researcher in designing the study and interpreting the outcomes. (Burns and Grove, 1993)

For more information on this very important research topic consult Chapter 4 by Marion Allison in this book and read the appropriate chapters in research text books e.g. Polit and Hungler (1991), or Treece and Treece (1986).

Having collected together, critically analysed and categorized a large body of literature concerning your area of interest it may become apparent that, despite there being a considerable body of research based knowledge available, nobody has published a concise, critical analysis of this topic. You may decide that rather than continuing through the remaining stages of the research process you would prefer to write an extensive literature review. If you are conducting your research as part of a degree programme check with your research supervisor that a major literature search is an acceptable alternative to data generation.

Many nursing libraries now have the computer facilities for users to conduct their own literature searches. All databases that are available for the searches have to be paid for by the library, therefore it is still advisable to consult a librarian as to other sources of literature concerning your field of interest. Try to think broadly: could useful articles be published in non-nursing journals?

Personally, I found the best way of identifying potentially useful articles was by consulting the reference lists of articles that I had already obtained. Libraries will always have a list of the journals that they take, and for which dates they have back editions of that journal available; this will tell you whether the article that you require is available at your local nursing library. Many libraries will also be able to tell you which local libraries take other journals that they do not stock themselves. Another useful source of journals is to consult local clinical specialists for the subjects that you are researching; in addition to any other advice that they may provide you with they may know somebody who has copies of the specialist journal that you are interested in seeing. This will almost certainly be quicker and cheaper than ordering articles via the library.

If you cannot find anyone who has a copy of the journal or article that you are interested in you will have to decide without seeing it if you want to pay the library to obtain a copy for you. Your library will be able to obtain a copy of any journal issue that has been ordered by the national library system and is still kept in storage by any library in the country, provided you give them the full reference of the article that you wish to obtain. Thus every journal published in the United Kingdom or in common use world wide is relatively easy to obtain. This process can take a long time and is expensive if you have to order many articles. If you are undertaking research as part of a college course you may be able to order a limited number of articles free from the college library, or your tutor may be able to order some for you.

Unfortunately, when undertaking the literature search for this research study I found that a large proportion of articles about The Health Belief Model and haemodialysis were published in American journals and the references that I obtained from articles concerning these topics proved extremely difficult to obtain (some articles that I thought might be useful arrived approximately a year after I ordered them from the library), and in many cases impossible to obtain in Britain.

I collected and critically evaluated literature concerning all of the six topics that I had previously identified (see Identifying the topic(s) to be researched) as being important in this particular study.

Having read each piece of literature carefully I wrote key words in a highlighter pen on the top of each article to remind me which topics were included in the article. I found that one-word reminders were best, e.g. when (the article included information on when patient education should be given); nurses (the article included information on nurses' perceptions of the importance of patients receiving information concerning different aspects of their treatment regime), etc. Most articles had more than one word clue written on them, and thus were potentially useful for inclusion in more than one section of the literature review chapter of my dissertation.

When an article had been coded it was added to one of the seven piles of articles, i.e. there was a pile for each of the six research topics and one for those that did not actually contain information relevant to this particular study but which I wanted to keep for potential future use (I had piles of articles all over my lounge floor for months!). I found this the best way of finding out if there were any areas of literature within the scope of my literature review for which I had insufficient data.

Consulting specialists in the field

Depending on the topic area that you decide to research into, and the research design that you plan to use, you may wish to consult a wide variety of specialists throughout the research process. As previously mentioned, for some researchers, meetings with clinical, educational or managerial colleagues may provide the initial idea for the research project, and thus they may be in a position to provide advice and support throughout the entire project.

In the planning stages of my research I consulted a number of specialists for advice and as part of my pilot study. Specialists you may wish to consult include:

1) Clinical specialists

    • For advice on content, methodology, clinical procedures/literature/ equipment, access to information and subjects, etc. They may also be willing to help create and pilot your research tools and are a useful source of appropriate literature.

    • Clinical colleagues working in related specialities provided me with some useful literature and were invaluable in piloting my research tools.

2) Research specialists

    • For advice on which method(s) to use, detailed advice on your chosen method(s), how to write a research proposal, how to obtain funding for your research, how to gain ethical approval, how to analyse and interpret your data, how to write up and submit your work for publication. They may also be willing to help create and pilot your research tools, and to help you collect and analyse your data. They are a useful source of information, and are familiar with literature on all aspects of the research process.

    • The hospital where I was working, and where I conducted my research, employed a research nurse. Part of her role was to support clinically based researchers throughout the whole research process. She helped me gain ethical approval for my study, and negotiated access to the consultants' computers to enable me to word process my dissertation at work in the evenings and at weekends.

    • My research supervisors were vital in providing the motivation to continue with my research. Discussions with them throughout the whole research process also helped me to ensure that the data that I collected were meaningful and interpreted fully in my dissertation.

3) Manufacturers' representatives

    • Most manufacturers that supply any part of the health service with commodities such as equipment, dressings, drugs, etc. have representatives that are employed to provide information and support for the users of their products. If you plan to conduct research involving their products the manufacturer's local representative is a useful source of advice about their products, and may lend or give you a supply of their product for use during your study. They should also be able to give you copies of previous studies carried out that involved their products. Remember that they are likely only to give you research that includes data favourable to their products. Manufacturers may also be a source of research funding or grants to present research at conferences.

4) Patients/relatives/carers

- Depending on the type of research planned, patients, relatives or carers who are not part of your chosen sample may be useful sources of advice, and are vital for conducting a pilot study (see Conducting a pilot study).
- A small group of patients piloted the research tools I had designed.

5) Statistician

- Students undertaking research as part of a college course will often have access to a statistician for advice on data analysis and significance. They may also offer advice on the creation of research tools that will make retrieval and analysis of data easier.
- I consulted one of the University of London's statisticians for conformation that I had chosen suitable statistical tests to analyse my data; it was confirmed that the discussion and conclusions of one of the research articles central to my literature review were flawed due to the use of an inappropriate statistical test.

6) Computer services

- Students undertaking research as part of a college course will often have access to a computer services department for advice on the creation of research tools that will make data retrieval and analysis easier. They can also provide education and resources to allow students to analyse their data using computers, which is vital when large amounts of data are being collected and analysed, and / or when complicated statistical analysis is required.

7) Other students/past students

- Peer support from other students who are undertaking or have undertaken your course is very important. The demoralizing feeling that you are the only person who has ever had a particular problem is most effectively counteracted by discussing your problems with somebody else who has experienced something similar. Other students may have already tackled the same problem that you are finding difficult, and thus can offer suggestions that may also work for you.

Talking with such specialists will often provide you with the initial idea for your research.

Considering the available resources and restraints

In beginning to plan your research project making a series of lists is helpful in clarifying your thoughts, e.g.

- Resource requirements – list everything that you can think of, e.g. your time, research assistant's time, secretarial support, statistical advice, photocopying, wordprocessing, travel costs, video camera, recorder.
- Breakdown of costs – for all of your resource requirements calculate their cost (some may be available to you for free). This will enable you to determine your funding needs.
- Timetable – in order to calculate funding needs a timetable of information such as length of time to be spent on data collection, data analysis, etc. is needed.
- Available resources – identify which of your resource requirements are readily available, e.g. colleagues may be willing to act as research assistants. This will enable you to determine which resources are not readily available and which you will have to pay for.
- Restraints – try to think of anything that you will have to organize or overcome in order to carry out your research. This list may act as a summary of the conclusions of your previous lists, e.g. funding needs, resource needs as well as a list of other barriers to be overcome, e.g. how will your family cope while you spend a lot of time completing your research project.

I carried out my research while being a university student and a full-time nurse, and I was lucky enough to be fully supported by both institutions throughout the process. This meant that I had relatively easy access to statisticians, wordprocessors, library facilities and photocopying.

There were two main restraints that I had to try and overcome: first, difficulty in obtaining relevant research articles – many of the articles that the librarians tried to obtain for me were published in American or Canadian journals that were not available in the UK; secondly, lack of personal time to carry out the research process – I was fortunate to be given one day a week study leave and to be allowed to use the wordprocessors at work in the evenings and at weekends. Without this help I would have found it much harder to keep to my timetable without paying for secretarial support. I was also fortunate to have the support of family and friends who were neglected for months at a time.

Writing a research proposal

A research proposal can be defined as 'a written summary of what the researcher intends to do, how and why' (Seaman and Verhonick, 1982). Parahoo and Reid (1988) extend this definition to include the questions where and when?

Research proposals are submitted when applying for funding, or ethical approval; the length and style of this proposal will be dictated by the body to whom it has to be sent. Thus depending upon the reason (s) why you are writing a research proposal your proposal may vary from a 400 word outline to a 3000 word detailed critique of the background to the study and description of the proposed research design.

Whatever its size it is usually necessary to include certain information if a research proposal is to be successful:

- the title of the research study;
- the theoretical background and rationale for the research study;
- the research questions / hypotheses to be tested by this research;
- details of the methods to be used for data generation and analysis;
- costs and proposed timetable for the stages of the research process;
- how the conclusions and recommendations of the study will be shared; and
- a reference list and glossary of terms used.

Obtaining ethical approval

Most research undertaken by nurses needs ethical approval before any data can be collected. Each health authority or trust has an ethical committee that is responsible for protecting the moral and ethical welfare of their patients. Thus anybody wishing to conduct research involving patients must apply to them for approval. Research projects involving staff, relatives or patients' records may also require approval from the local ethics committee; if in doubt contact the secretary to the committee for advice. Research projects involving staff or students of any college or school will require approval from the management of that institution.

Each individual ethics committee has its own application procedure that may include any or all of the following: an application form; submission of a research proposal; interview with a committee member; and appearance at an ethics committee meeting. Some committees have the system whereby small-scale research projects are initially vetted by the secretary to the committee or some sub-committee who can give chairman's approval to studies that involve no ethical issues that require the consideration of the full ethics committee.

Research projects that have not been carefully planned, are not well presented, and proposals that lack sufficient information will be discarded by the ethics committee, together with those that are unethical. In order to promote your chances of gaining ethical approval take advice from people who have already gained approval from your ethics committee, talk to members of the committee (the secretary or clinical representatives are often willing to help aspiring nurse researchers), and find out if there are any local research nurses who would be willing to give you advice.

Don't be to downhearted if at first your application isn't successful. Read carefully any explanation that you are given as to why your research has not been given ethical approval. If you still don't understand what you have to do to receive approval write to the chairman and ask for clarification or an appointment to discuss your unsuccessful application. Think carefully about any changes that the committee is asking you to make to your study before it will give you ethical approval. You will not receive approval without these changes; so if you feel that your research will not be possible in the light of the suggested changes you will have completely to rethink your research design (see Figure 2.1).

Many studies are given ethical approval providing minor changes are made. Often the changes asked for are small, such as the addition, rewording or removal of a question from a questionnaire. Remember that even if you are convinced that your wording of the question was much clearer than that of the board's question, your wording was not given ethical approval and you must only use the version that they have approved.

Ethical approval was necessary for my proposed research project since it involved using questionnaires with both staff and patients. I was fortunate that the hospital's research nurse helped me to complete my application form and that, as a member of the ethics committee, she sponsored my research project at the committee meeting. Thus I was able to submit an application to the ethics committee that was successful, without revision, at the first attempt.

Applying for funding

In my experience many nurses meet all of the costs of their own research themselves rather than applying for funding. This may be because traditionally nursing research tends to be small-scale clinical studies that can be carried out by one researcher for minimal expense. Another possible reason is that in general nurses do not know who they can apply to for funding for their research. Applying for funding can also be very time consuming and costly if you have to send a number of copies of a large research proposal and application form to several potential sources of funding. Many funding bodies will also expect the applicant to attend a panel interview, and if granted funding, to present their findings at a later meeting. I suspect that, for a number of these reasons, nurses choose not to apply for funding. Personally having calculated my research costs, having deducted the cost of anything that my employers or the university were supplying, I decided that it was not worth spending a lot of time and effort seeking funding for this small amount.

Sources of funding for research are limited, but, as nursing research is becoming more recognized as research of a quality comparable with that produced by doctors, more sources of funding are becoming available. In fact Burns and Grove (1993) report that some of the available money is currently not being used, leading funding bodies to conclude that nurses do not need research funding.

For clinical research that will be of direct benefit to the researcher's employing organization that organization may be able to provide the necessary funding. Medical charities and pharmaceutical / medical equipment companies are worth approaching if your research is concerned with their particular interests. Some hospitals and universities have research grants available to past and presents students or employees. Your trade union, local nurses union or League of Friends are also worth approaching as sources of funding. Other funding bodies offer scholarships and specific awards that are advertised nationally in the nursing press e.g. *The Nursing Times* and *The Nursing Standard*. Your local nursing or University library should have copies of guides such as *Directory of Grant Making Trusts*, published by Charities Aid Foundation, *Grants Register*, published by Macmillan, and *Handbook of British Medical Charities*, published by the Association of Medical Charities.

Identifying/constructing the instruments

A research instrument is any piece of equipment (e.g. sphygmomanometer) or written tool (e.g. questionnaire) that is used to collect research data. The reliability and validity of these instruments is important if meaningful data are to be collected. If you can use instruments already in use and already tested for reliability and validity this will save you a lot of time and effort. It also aids comparison with other researcher's work. If designing your own research tools these issues must be considered before they are used to collect data (for advice on reliability and validity consult any of the numerous books on research methodology available at your local college or hospital library).

The instruments that I used within this research were a combination of questionnaires to determine the current level of patient knowledge concerning different aspects of their treatment regimen and compliance, and Likert type scales to measure the perceptions of patients and nurses as to the importance of patients receiving information concerning their treatment regimen. Since none of these instruments was already available I had to write them all myself. In order to do this I consulted a number of books on research methodology (e.g. Fox, 1982; Polit and Hungler, 1991), critiqued articles on compliance and haemodialysis treatment, discussed their content with colleagues, and piloted the instruments with clinical colleagues and patients.

Consulting the key people

Depending on the type of research that you propose doing you may identify key people you need to consult to gain access to subjects, equipment, or other facilities. Gaining ethical approval to question patients who come into hospital does not automatically mean that the consultant of these patients will also give you permission to conduct a study on their patients, or that the ward manager will grant you access. Send all of these key people a copy of your research proposal and consent from the ethics committee, together with a letter requesting their permission to carry out your study. They may wish to discuss the proposal with you, and will certainly expect to receive a copy of your research report and to discuss the findings and implications with you after your research has been completed.

By referring to the research process framework (see Research process) it is clear that it can be to your advantage to consult the key people you have identified at any of the stages at which you wish to use resources under their control, e.g. you need access to a clinical area to conduct a pilot study.

Having discussed my research ideas with the unit manager prior to writing the research proposal and the fact that one of the consultants was the chairman of the ethics committee meant that gaining permission to carry out the study was relatively easy. Consulting with the research nurse throughout the whole process promoted communication concerning the progress of my research.

Conducting a pilot study

For many researchers an important planning stage is conducting a pilot study. A pilot study is a small-scale version of the main study. It is conducted to test the research methodology and the validity of research instruments. Pilot studies allow problems and limitations to be identified and corrected before the main study is carried out. Thus a pilot study is conducted after all the necessary research instruments have been identified or constructed and is included in the research proposal submitted to gain ethical approval for the study (see Writing a research proposal).

An aspect of conducting a pilot study that is often forgotten is that a pilot study can also be used to test the mechanisms by which data are to be collected, e.g. how questionnaires are distributed, and completed questionnaires collected, and the effectiveness / cost of methods that could be used to promote response rate. For more information see Chapter 4.

Because I had to construct all of the instruments used to collect data in this research study it was important to conduct a pilot study to test these instruments. Because there were instruments to collect data from both patients and staff the instruments had to be piloted by groups of both staff and patients that were similar to but not part of the chosen sample. To pilot the patients' instruments I used the patients receiving haemodialysis at a separate satellite dialysis unit, and the staff questionnaires were piloted by staff working with patients in renal failure who were being treated by CAPD or transplantation.

Altering the design/instruments

After the data have been collected in the pilot study it may be necessary to alter the design of the proposed study or amend the instruments. Changes may be needed for a number of reasons, e.g. the pilot study demonstrated that when collected data were analysed, additional data were required from each subject in order for them to be meaningful; questionnaires were found to contain questions that were ambiguous, contained double negatives, duplicated data collection, contained double-barrelled questions, contained questions that asked for information that the subjects felt was too personal or too confidential, etc.

Desirable changes in design or instrumentation may be minor, e.g. deleting an unnecessary point from your observation guide, or major, e.g. adding relatives to your list of subjects to be interviewed. Minor changes to both instruments and design can be made without further consultation with the ethics committee, (if you are not sure that the changes you need to make are minor, consult the secretary to the ethics committee that gave you ethical approval). Major changes must always receive approval from the ethics committee. This does not mean that you will have to submit a new research proposal to the ethics committee, but that you will need to write to the chairperson of the ethics committee reminding him/her of your approved study and explaining in detail how you wish to amend or extend the approved study, and why. Unless your changes suggest potential ethical problems the chairperson will write to you to give his/her approval for the changes to the study.

Following the pilot study I had a major change to make to my research design, and minor changes to make to one of the instruments.

As previously stated (see Identifying the topic(s) to be researched), after I had gained ethical approval I decided to extend my study to include data on patient compliance. In order to collect these data from the patients' records I also needed ethical approval for this part of the study. This was gained by applying to the chairperson of the ethics committee for his/her approval to extend an already approved project. Because compliance was obviously closely linked to the rest of my study, and my methodology did not suggest any ethical problems this approval was readily given. If I had had to wait until after the next ethics committee my data collection would have been delayed by 6–8 weeks.

Collecting the data

In order to write your research proposal you will have to decide how you are going to collect your data. As previously stated (see Writing a research proposal) planning how you are going to collect your data does not just mean that, for example, you are going to use a questionnaire; it also means deciding how those questionnaires are going to be distributed to your sample, how you will attempt to promote the response rate and what your time scale is for collecting your data.

I collected data from both patients and staff using questionnaires and Likert type scales (for more information on scales and questionnaires see research methodology books such as Oppenheim, 1992 or Burns and Grove, 1993).

Analysing the data

As part of your research proposal (see Writing a research proposal) you will probably have already decided exactly how you are going to analyse your data. The methods you use will almost always be dictated by the methodology you have chosen, therefore if you do not want to analyse your data statistically, do not write a research design that only yields useful data when the information is tested statistically.

Some data analysis is normally done by hand, e.g. quantitative data analysis where groups and themes are identified before looking for links between these groups (for more detail on qualitative data analysis see research methodology books such as Burns and Grove, 1993). Although I analysed my data using statistical tests I performed these all by hand because of the relatively small numbers in each of my sample groups (29 patients and 10 staff) and because this was less time consuming than travelling to the university to use the computers to analyse my data.

For large studies or where very complicated statistical tests are required analysis usually requires access to computer facilities. All universities will have these facilities available to their students, together with computer staff who will teach and advise students on the use of appropriate statistical software. These facilities may be available to other researchers via the university's research division.

Writing the report

The way that you choose to write your report will mainly depend upon the reason why you are writing the report, i.e. who it is aimed at. A funding body, research interest group or clinical organization will expect a brief written report (see Sharing the findings) whereas a university will require that your research is presented as a dissertation when the research has been carried out as part of a degree programme.

In my case my research report took the form of a dissertation since I was required to submit this to the university in order to gain my MSc in Nursing. A dissertation is a very large piece of work (mine was approximately 20 000 words) consisting of an extensive critical review of relevant literature, a description of the methods of data generation and analysis, a presentation and discussion of the results and a conclusion that summarizes the research and includes the researcher's recommendations. Each University will have its own rules as to how they require research reports to be presented.

Sharing the findings

This is the stage of the research process that researchers often forget exists. A research study is incomplete if the findings and recommendations are not made available for use.

There are a variety of ways in which a researcher can share his/her findings, e.g. writing an article for publication in a journal, or contributing to a book of similar work. Research can also reach an interested audience if it is presented at an appropriate conference, study day, or interest group. Another way of sharing work is to present a seminar based upon the research to fellow researchers and clinical colleagues. A written summary of the research, its findings, and recommendations should also be given to any funding body involved with the project and to any clinical organization or group of colleagues that participated in the research; they may also expect you to present your research to them personally.

Sharing your findings and recommendations with clinical organizations and colleagues is particularly important because they are the people most likely to wish to benefit practically from your work. It is also a way of thanking them for participating in or helping you with your research. This feedback will act as an encouragement for the next time somebody wishes to conduct research in this clinical area. It may be you!

On reflection this was by far the weakest stage of the research process for me. I prepared a seminar based upon my research for my colleagues as part of the ongoing staff development programme within the unit. I also discussed some of my findings informally with appropriate colleagues, e.g. the unit's dietitian. The fact that soon after completing this research the unit moved to another hospital, and that I changed jobs very soon after this move meant that it was not possible to use my results to help the patients in the way that I had hoped. Until now I haven't published anything from the research that I carried out to gain my MSc in Nursing. I now more fully appreciate the importance of this stage of the research process.

Conclusion

A number of my research students have complained that they find research books dull and unreadable. Unfortunately in some cases they are right, and useful information is not conveyed to potential users. I have tried to write this chapter in a way that shares advice and information with its readers without becoming boring or patronizing. It contains research tips and suggestions that I have collected throughout my time as a nurse researcher, research student, and currently as a research supervisor and educator. I have found many of them useful and I am always pleased to receive further hints that I can use myself and share with my research students.

Research should be an interesting and educational experience both for the researchers and their readers. The research process can provide a framework to aid understanding for both groups if the information is available so that everyone can understand the necessity for the research, the processes that the researcher has to go through to complete each separate stage of the research process, and the ways in which each stage fits together. I hope that this chapter has provided useful insights for novice and experienced researchers and their readers.

References

Burns N & Grove S K (1993) *The Practice of Nursing Research: Conduct, Critique and Utilization,* 2nd edn. W B Saunders, Philadelphia.

Fox D J (1982) *Fundamentals of Research in Nursing,* 4th edn. Appleton-Century-Crofts, Norwalk, CT.

Goddard H A & Powers M J (1982) Educational needs of patients undergoing haemodialysis: a comparison of patient and nurse perceptions. *Dialysis and Transplantation* 11 (7): 578–583.

Herbert M (1990) *Planning a Research Project: A Guide for Practitioners and Trainees in the Helping Professions.* Cassell, London.

Janz N K and Becker M H (1984) The health belief model a decade later. *Health Education Quarterly* 11 (1) 1–47.

Oppenheim A N (1992) *Questionnaire Design, Interviewing and Attitude Measurement,* 2nd edn. Pinter, London.

Parahoo K and Reid N (1988) Research skills 3: writing a research proposal. *Nursing Times* 84 (41) 49–52.

Polit D F and Hungler B P (1991) *Nursing Research: Principles and Methods,* 4th edn. Lippincott, Philadelphia.

Reddecliffe G M (1991) An examination of the educational needs and treatment knowledge of hospital-based haemodialysis patients and how these relate to compliance. Unpublished MSc thesis, University of London.

Reid N G & Boore J R P (1987) *Research Methods and Statistics in Health Care.* Edward Arnold, London.

Seaman C H C and Verhonick P J (1982) *Research Methods for Undergraduate Students in Nursing.* Appleton-Century-Crofts, Norwalk, CT.
Treece E W and Treece J W (1986) *Elements of Research In Nursing,* 4th edn. Mosby, St Louis.

Glossary of terms

Continuous ambulatory peritoneal dialysis (CAPD)

Treatment performed by a person with ESRF to correct that person's electrolyte, fluid and acid–base imbalance. This treatment is based upon the ability of the patient's peritoneum to act as a semi-permeable membrane across which waste products can diffuse. Every day the patient drains sterile CAPD fluid onto the outer layer of their peritoneum via a permanent CAPD catheter. This fluid remains inside the patient for a few hours to allow diffusion of waste products to occur. The fluid is then drained out and replaced with another bag of CAPD fluid. The patient normally performs this exchange procedure 4–6 times every day depending upon his/her individual treatment regimen.

End stage renal failure (ESRF)

This is reached when less than 10 per cent of a person's normal kidney function remains; it is incompatible with life (Reddecliffe, 1991).

Haemodialysis

Treatment performed on the blood of a person in ESRF to correct that person's electrolyte, fluid and acid–base imbalance. This is performed by pumping the patient's blood, via the dialysis tubing, past a semi-permeable membrane and back to the patient. At the same time dialysate is pumped past the other side of the semi-permeable membrane. Exchange occurs across the membrane so that the 'cleaned' blood returning to the patient is more 'normally' balanced; water is removed from the patient at the same time (Reddecliffe, 1991).

3

A case in point:
teaching nurse teachers

Sally Thomson

This chapter in particular:

- *clarifies a case study approach to research and explores some of the considerations around it;*
- *explores ethical issues surrounding this work from a personal perspective;*
- *uses a reflective approach to research explicitly in journal keeping and implicitly in the written style;*
- *refers to supervision as a supportive process;*
- *is written in the case study style;*
- *uses tables to mix qualitative and quantative data.*

Introduction

This chapter has two themes. First, it describes a case study approach to research, followed by a discussion of the development of an ethical code of conduct. It then moves on to present aspects of the case study in order to highlight aspects of the introductory debate and also to share research findings. During the chapter I discuss, where appropriate, events which triggered personal learning, difficulties and how problems were solved. It clearly shows the fallibility of the researcher and, like the other chapters, is a reflective account.

The case study examined the effects of preparation upon the classroom teaching strategies that student teachers adopted during teaching practice and one year after completion of nurse teacher training.

Teacher preparation was carried out on two sites, during the course at the educational institution and the colleges of nursing that provided teaching practice placements.

In order to be true to case study ideals and to give a flavour of how such a research approach materializes, I have chosen to focus in depth upon two aspects of the study, that is, the college lecturers and the process of assessing teaching. To give some clarity to the study, a brief discription is given of teaching practice and how students are prepared by the college for this event. To demonstrate the complexity of the nature of teaching, some of the influences that affect teaching strategies are explored briefly.

The case study as an approach to educational research

A case study format was adopted for this piece of research. This approach has been described as 'the examination of an instance in action' (Walker, 1980). It reveals biography, personality intentions and values. Stenhouse (1975) claims the approach is 'strong in reality', permitting the researcher to discover the uniqueness of the field situation. The flexibility and freedom of a case study, its nature and method is favoured by Simons (1981). It is also a systematic, scientific approach (Nisbett and Watt, 1978), allowing for the probing and analysis of its 'multifarious phenomena' (Cohen and Manion, 1985). Case studies provide a rich source of hypotheses, and display individual events within a total network of relationships, demonstrating links (Treece and Treece, 1982). This latter point is important as it means that a study can be started on almost any relevant theme at any point in time. The problem I experienced was that of knowing when to stop. The more links I discovered, the more it became apparent that other avenues needed to be explored and stopping became a problem.

Case study evidence alerts teachers to factors which may affect their work (Stenhouse, 1984). It enables an informed judgement to be made prior to a course of action. It allows teachers to see behind what is taken for granted, removing the flattening effect of habit (Ruddock, 1985). It was hoped that the work would provide guidance for the curriculum development of a new course for nurse teachers. Fortunately, the method lends itself to a researcher working alone (Nisbett and Watt, 1978).

The issue of generalization has been debated by many writers in educational research (Stenhouse, 1975; Gage, 1978; Nisbett and Watt, 1978; Cohen and Manion, 1985). My intention was that the study would be illuminative and allow the transfer of successful practices, whether carried out intentionally or intuitively, from one course of teacher preparation to another.

Problems in a case study undoubtedly arise from the researcher working in a familiar situation. Burgess (1984) questions whether the 'native' will be able to recognize patterns and elucidate meanings in events. He points to the problems inherent within the relationship between investigator and informant, and in occupying the dual role of teacher and researcher. Treece and Treece (1982) predict the likelihood of researcher subjectivity within the context of social involvement such as exists, causing misjudgements of both depth and insight. Woods (1985) cautions that immersion within a culture may block theory construction. '... It is impossible to clear one's mind when working in one's own culture or close to it' (Walker, 1980). Pollard (1985) offers a useful strategy to overcome, or climb out of, a cultural immersion. He relates how, despite 'going native' within a school, he kept a degree of detachment in his mind.

Lofland (1971) advises researchers to publish the degree of specificity regarding the context under study. During my preparatory reading, a research model evolved the style of which was influenced by Bennett (1976). Figure 3.1 is a representation of the research process. The proposal was flexible and allowed for adaptations as the process developed. Parlett and Hamilton (1972) advocate a specific ground rule of cross checking data, clearly spelling out the criteria for rejection and selection of material. Additionally, Lofland (1971) suggests that subjectivity can be overcome if the researcher details how the study was conducted, how and why decisions were made to collect data, how cooperation was secured from participants, and how the relationship with the latter was developed. He also advocates a confession of the 'social blunders' committed by the researcher, and the services provided in return for data. This advice was internalized by myself. Further influenced by Lofland (1971), I kept an ongoing diary of the research experience, including, as he suggests, private feelings about the setting, emotions aroused and difficulties encountered. This diary became a significant resource, listening to my neurotic outpourings as well as logging the highs, lows, confusions and visions of the study. I carried it with me wherever I went. Often in the night I would switch on the light, scribble a few lines of inspiration and return to sleep, knowing my ideas would not be lost by the morning. Indeed, many of these jottings were relative brainwaves! It certainly helped me to manage my emotional involvement in this study.

In the light of the above considerations, I selected a case study approach to investigate my own place of work. I believed the enquiry did not lend itself to hard statistical data. My intention was to portray the factors which influenced student teachers' classroom teaching strategies.

The ethical issues surrounding the case study

Regardless of the intention, a case study may damage people, organizations and reputations (Nisbett and Watt, 1978). Therefore, I tried to incorporate a variety of techniques and perspectives into the study, to increase reliability and to reduce the harm that an incident portrayed in isolation might cause. Treece and Treece (1982) comment on the difference in case studies designed to research undesirable traits, as opposed to strengths, which

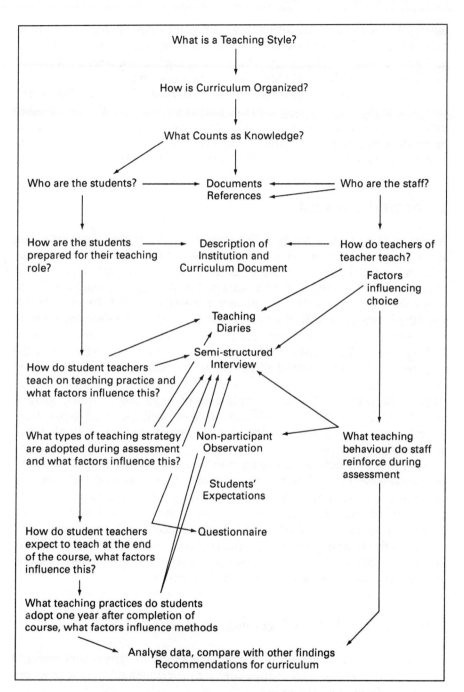

Figure 3.1 Does preparation influence classroom teaching strategies?

emerge in the results. The former may cause considerable harm. The intention of this work was to demystify and make explicit the positive lecturer and institutional influences upon the developing teacher, with the intention of adopting the successful ploys into a new programme.

This section outlines the ethical code of conduct adhered to during and after the study, highlighting areas of particular concern. The stand taken details a way of life which reflects my personal values. The source of imperative originates from the codes, practices and reflections of others, which complements and elaborates on my own thinking.

Informed consent

Adelman (1981) acknowledges the need for rules when generating case study data to control the acquisition and use of information.

In order to obtain informed consent, I offered an explanation of the research, and the nature of, and reasons for, the study. Participants were given the option to withdraw at any time (Treece and Treece, 1982). I sought an interview with the Director of Education to gain permission to study my workplace. This was readily given. But, at a later date, I learned a sharp lesson. I had asked if it was necessary to write and confirm the discussion, and was grateful to hear that it would not be needed. Some months later, the same person, in a harrassed moment, denied any knowledge of the research. It was a simple case of forgetting. A quick 'ground smoothing' operation followed and all was well. A short letter from myself summarizing the meeting would have prevented a hugh surge of adrenaline!

Burgess (1984) outlines a situation in which the researcher may not be sure of whether the information is useful or not. If I was doubtful about the use of data, I included it within the transcripts returned to participants. This enabled them to make a decision as to whether or not they would consent to its use, or wished to edit certain aspects of the dialogue.

The methods and procedures utilized were made explicit and clearly visible in order to remove the threat of covert activity, especially for colleagues who had a researcher/peer in their midst.

Confidentiality and access to data

'People own the facts of their lives and have a right to deny others access to them' (Walker, 1980). Walker stipulates that confidentiality must be a continuous methodological concern.

The college and course under scrutiny are well known in nursing circles, as are many of my colleagues. Burgess (1984) discovered that there is no foolproof way of protecting people. In his study, he relates how people were easily identified by those 'in the know'. This was one of my main concerns. Burgess reflects that it might be advisable to change the name of the course and personnel. He recommends adopting pseudonyms that have a logical relationship to the name, but not changing the gender of the participants. These measures were adopted in the study. The institution was not named and all participants, the course and validating university were given pseudonyms. Despite this, I recognized that elements of the study might be identifiable and participants were made aware of this.

Pring (1984) offers useful advice in suggesting how the researcher may establish a relationship of trust with those researched. He holds that this could be achieved by clarifying the kinds of knowledge sought. He debates the ethical dilemma of the right to know and the right of confidentiality, contending that the researcher is obliged to show the interpretation of data, and to be open to cross-examination by the group researched. Finally, he holds that any replies of those researched are incorporated into the findings. Before embarking on any strategies, I held briefing meetings with the groups concerned to facilitate free exchange.

Pring (1984) further advises the researcher to seek a balance between the private and public interests of the work. He warns of the political significance of institutions being studied and the interests of authorities. I considered that those reading the case study might have differing motivations and questions from the researcher, and be seeking answers to a different set of questions. Nisbett and Watt (1978) suggest that the published comments, criticisms and replies of those researched may be helpful in expressing a point a better way, and so further illuminate the study.

Walker (1980) discusses the perceptions of the researched. He indicates that the researcher may be viewed as a conspirator if he/she interviews students and does not reveal the data. Conversely, staff may see the researcher as 'God-like', which may strain relationships and he suggests that staff often exert considerable pressure on the researcher to 'tell all!'. He contends that the researcher must resolve such conflicts. My experience certainly was not one of feeling 'God-like'. The conflict I experienced was not generated by the three lecturers under scrutiny, who seemed to go out of their way to put me at ease, but from my peer group not being researched, who often commented on the intrusive nature of my methodology.

Walker also discusses the pressure arising from various interest groups and I did experience pressure to reveal what was going on.

Simons (1981) reflects that principles of procedure protect the researched from misuse of data. The use of all data in this study was negotiated with informants who made the ultimate decision as to whether or not it could be used. During this interaction, I was careful also to check my perception of events against those of the participants.

Protection from injury

Subjects must be assured protection against physical, social or emotional injury (Treece and Treece, 1982) or from any consequent harm arising from participating in the study (RCN, 1977). Walker (1980) cautions that the case study is a selected measure of events in which the researcher's interpretation of situations cannot account for the perception of others. He suggests that the misuse of data must be carefully predicted. I would hope that my concern with the people and place under study have added a protective veneer to the work.

Scott (1985) elaborates upon the power relationships at work during the process of research, especially when working with peers, when confidentiality poses a problem. The dual role of friend and researcher may be jeopardized, but this ambiguity can be resolved by reporting back to those concerned (Pollard, 1985).

Burgess (1984) discusses current research and identifies the 'guilty knowledge' that this may generate for the investigator, as if one knows something one should not. On the whole, my research was an overt, formal collection of data, and I tried to step in and out of the researcher/colleague/lecturer role. This was not always easy; indeed, eavesdropping was often illuminative and influenced my study. Permission, however, was always sought to use information gleaned in this way.

Researcher skills

It is the researcher's responsibility to possess the knowledge and skills compatible with the demands of the investigation (RCN, 1977), while not overstepping the boundaries of confidence (Treece and Treece, 1982). The researcher should also acknowledge personal limitations and lack of detachment from the area of study. Additionally, the way his/her presence may have affected the areas under scrutiny should always be stated (RCN, 1977).

Lofland (1971) reflects upon the difficulties of maintaining neutrality, and he suggests that a moral study rests upon loyalty to the researched. He describes the 'seductive effect' of personal involvement and of coming to like the researched. I thought carefully about Lofland's ideas in which he seems to describe a 'them and us' situation. It might have applied in this context as I investigated my work culture and colleagues, but I entered into the work with relationships already firmly established.

One of the crucial skills of the researcher is reporting the truth. Patton (1980) suggests that the reporter's perspective is the truth. He finds speculations on casual relationships entirely appropriate, as long as the speculative nature is clearly apparent. He holds that researcher effects tend to be overrated, but advises the researcher to keep a balance between the objective and subjective elements.

The ethical issues surrounding an investigation of one's workplace are complex and the implications far reaching. The experience and advice of the writers mentioned helped me to think through a code of conduct with an awareness of the dangers and difficulties inherent within research practice. Additionally, I worked closely with my supervisor who had a duty to ensure the methodology adopted was valid and acceptable.

The code selected provided a way of behaving which rested upon respect for those who cooperated to help me search for answers. Aspects of the work caused me feelings of vulnerability and adherence to an ethical code helped my adaptation to this stressor.

Nevertheless, my diary and discussion upon completing the study reflected the discomfort associated with the case study approach and having to investigate the world of colleagues, friends and peers. These are people whom I admire and hold in high esteem, and who frequently act as my role models. For those who helped in the study, the research placed a considerable increase in workload, imposing upon heavily overstretched work schedules. There were times when, because of this, I experienced considerable vulnerability and unease. I suspected that I was often frustrating the work and personal needs of others while seeking information to meet my own.

In addition to the above, it was often difficult to work critically at my own place of work, since during my time there I have come to internalize many of its attitudes and values. I often felt that I was very alone conducting my investigation, as it was not possible to share my emotions. My research supervisor therefore was often used as a sounding board.

Pollard (1985) suggests that the necessary degree of detachment is difficult to achieve and I would agree with this. Two events particularly stand out in my mind as fraught. On the first occasion I made a particularly tactless remark in front of John Barnes (pseudonym), a colleague, about the course; it was the day before I was due to go out with him on a teaching assessment. I wished I could have fallen through the floor at my stupidity! The second occasion arose when I had arranged to meet the three lecturers involved in the research, to brief them for some data collection. John asked me to delay the meeting for five minutes, and when we finally got together, the three were preoccupied with concerns about their work.

I felt very aware both of my needs to obtain their help and of their needs to survive the working day. I felt a nuisance. My feelings of incompetence were enhanced when I invited them to choose the pseudonym for the college and the course, and they questioned my strategy for making the two anonymous. It was a small incident, but it shook me, I think, because of how quickly I felt deskilled. In retrospect, of course, I should have left them to continue with their work. I believe a 'pay off' (Lofland, 1971) was offered to the lecturers when I took on the teaching commitments of one of them during a period of planned surgery and convalescence. The 'pay off' for the student group was small. They gave willingly of their free time during a rigorous and demanding course of study. I wrote a letter of thanks, and circulated a small summary of the study, but it seemed a paltry reward.

It was also difficult to assess how much impact my presence had upon the student teacher and assessor during non-participant observation. I felt it was minimal (but this may have been my perceptual set!). The students who were invited knew me quite well. Several had experience of me acting as a clinical teaching assessor from a previous course and seemed to welcome me quite literally with open arms. My colleagues similarly seemed unperturbed by my presence. Each seemed natural and relaxed, and acted as I predicted they might (again I may have seen what I expected).

I think my own evaluation of the observation technique might have been different if the teaching sessions had not been so successful. I was privileged to be party to five outstanding student performances, and I think it may have been a difficult role to exercise in a 'near miss' situation.

An ethical code of conduct can offer crucial principles that direct research practice. In reality other factors may mean that one is less honourable than one intends to be, for example, your own need to keep to your research timetable.

The three lecturers under scrutiny

John Barnes is course tutor to the Nurse Teachers Diploma course. He joined the college and began this role in 1982. He started his nursing career in the Royal Air Force and commenced his teaching experience there in an unqualified capacity in 1977. Upon completion of the Sister Tutors Diploma course he returned to the RAF, taking charge of a school of nursing as a senior tutor which prepared pupil nurses for enrolment. When the school of nursing closed, John worked as a 'Nursing Process Change Agent and Coordinator' in a 'peripatetic role', covering all RAF hospitals. During that time, he also lectured at a local college of further education to Diploma in Nursing students, teaching psychology and physiology. In 1981, he obtained a Diploma in Education, and in 1983 completed his MA (Ed.) in Curriculum Studies.

Over and above his current role, John has many professional commitments. He is an external examiner for Barchester University for teaching practice assessment, and a member of the same institution's Review Group for the Nurse Teachers Diploma. Additionally, he is a member of a National Board design working group, preparing resource materials for nurse teachers. John is also a critical reader for the psychology units of the Diploma in Nursing by distance learning, and teaches special topics in educational psychology and curriculum studies to MA and Diploma in Education students at the University of Barchester. He is described by one of his colleagues as

> an enthusiastic, outgoing person, interested in everything, and more than willing to play his part in new developments. He is a colleague one can rely upon, hardworking and ready to share his expertise. His sense of humour helps him to keep things in perspective, and he is invariably even tempered. His devotion to physical fitness is an example to us all!
>
> John is a conscientious teacher, who plans well in advance for all his commitments. His knowledge is up-to-date, and is used imaginatively. John enjoys a good relationship with the students, creating a safe collegial partnership in learning for them. He is innovative in his teaching methods, and has very good organizational ability which facilitates the smooth running of courses for which he is responsible. He is always supportive towards students and colleagues.

John commented on how pleased he was with the reference, and felt he could 'identify with it'. He describes his role in terms of having overall responsibility for the administrative aspects of the course. His teaching commitment to the course is primarily educational psychology, but he also 'dips into curriculum studies, sharing some materials with Claire Honeycutt', in a team-teaching format. He also teaches some aspects of the research process.

He describes his teaching style as 'student-centred', and relates how he analyses the way in which he can achieve the goals of the session by maximizing upon student participation and minimizing his overt participation: 'I go into any session with that formula in mind'. John describes his teaching approach as informal, informative and humorous: 'it seems a contradiction in terms, but it's structured in a laid-back way'.

He reflects upon how his teaching approach has developed to become more flexible and he feels he is more able to adapt sessions to the students' needs:

> I've developed that since being here. I take a lot more risks now. If it doesn't work out then I don't worry about it so much, I'm a lot more comfortable with not having high control.

His teaching style has evolved from reading, watching others

> and constantly thinking how can I do this differently to make it more enjoyable for the group, for two reasons. Firstly, I want to develop my repertoire of teaching, skills and, secondly, to model a range of skills for the students.

He operates his teaching from the findings of social learning theories, and feels that a teacher needs to be credible in knowledge and expertise and hopefully humanistic, warm, and effective. John additionally runs a weekly aerobic class for students and staff at the college. He has contributed several chapters on educational psychology to books on nursing and education, and is currently preparing a book on the same subject.

The co-tutor to the Nurse Teacher's Diploma is Claire Honeycutt (pseudonym), who also joined the college in 1982 as a lecturer. Claire teaches Principles and Practice of Education to the Nurse Teacher's Diploma. Claire began her nursing career as a registered general nurse and moved on to qualify as a sick children's nurse and midwife. She obtained her Midwife Teacher's Diploma in 1974. Since that time, Claire's teaching career has focused upon midwifery, with four years spent as the assistant principal of a midwife teacher training college. She obtained a Bachelor of Humanities by full-time study during that period. Additionally, Claire is an external examiner for Barchester University for teaching practice assessments, and has published articles in nursing journals. In 1987, Claire completed her MA (Education) in Curriculum Studies. Claire is described in the following way:

> a refined, cheerful person, who readily establishes a rapport with people. She is highly intelligent, quick-witted, and possesses an excellent sense of humour which helps her to keep the demands of working in the college in perspective. She is invariably even-tempered, which makes her such an ideal colleague to work with on a day-to-day basis.
>
> Claire is a conscientious person who is very popular with the students. She has the ability to select material and plan it at just the right level whenever she teaches. Her organisational abilities are excellent, though casual visitors to the office might puzzle about this on a first glance at her desk top!
>
> I know that Claire is the best person I have ever worked with (or am likely to) and consider myself to be privileged to have had the pleasure of working with her over the past five and a half years! Her students think the world of her, and so do all our colleagues at the college, I suspect.

Claire believes that teaching and learning activities should be 'fun': 'if people feel they've learned something and enjoyed it as well, I'm delighted; my relationship with the group is "very important"'. She describes herself as 'susceptible to vibes' from the students: 'if we're all on the same wavelength, it makes life much easier, in terms of rapport'.

She claims that she is an unscientific person who has a tendency to believe that teaching is an art. She describes her teaching style as 'democratic', giving students a choice with the process of learning: 'but I regard the content as mostly essential. I'm reasonably adaptable – if people are flagging, we stop, if possible'.

Claire describes how her teaching strategies have evolved from exchange of ideas with John:

> something rubs off, but it's more unconscious . . . I've used much more variety in teaching methods since I came here, probably in part because of the nature of the subject matter.

The Principal Lecturer to the teaching courses is Ruth Copeman (pseudonym). John and Claire who share an office are both members of her team. Ruth, with John and Claire, shares the bulk of the teaching upon the course in question. Her commitment is to the area of 'Human Relationships', part of which involves a cooperative teaching venture with two other lecturers. Ruth's career began in general nursing, and she studied midwifery before embarking upon her teaching career. She moved from clinical teacher to senior tutor at a London teaching hospital before joining the college as a lecturer in 1979. Prior to John Barnes' appointment, Ruth acted as a course tutor to the Nurse Teacher's Diploma and became a principal lecturer in 1981. Ruth has a BA (Hons) degree in Psychology with Social Anthropology and an MSc in Occupational Behaviour. Additionally, she has completed a part-time course in Pastoral Care and Counselling.

Her colleague described her in the following way:

> As a person, Ruth is warm, sensitive and generous, and has a very attractive smile. Supportive when necessary, she is adept at judging the best sort of support needed. She is more of a listener than a talker and would most certainly respect confidences. She seems also to have a delightful affinity and sympathy for more individualistic or slightly eccentric people! She is intelligent, conscientious and hard-working, and her organization is meticulous.
>
> The above qualities suggest to me that, as a teacher, Ruth's preparation is thorough, with the ability to facilitate a safe and non-threatening learning environment. She is perceptive to the needs of individuals. I see her as being particularly skilled in handling group discussions and sessions involving experiential learning, and also in helping students to develop these skills themselves and feel positive about them.

Ruth, along with John, is also a member of the course curriculum review group. She has recently resigned as Chief Assessor to one of the units of the Diploma in Nursing and external examiner to the BA Nursing Studies degree of the National University of Ireland in Dublin. She is also a member of a variety of committees at a school of nursing and national level. She has had several papers published.

Ruth perceives teaching and learning as a partnership, and describes how she negotiates the human relationship aspects of the curriculum with the students. She attributes her approach to teaching as part of her

> total approach to life, that is respect for other persons. I try to maintain that always in the way I handle students and teaching sessions. If you get that right, a lot of other things happen in the best possible way anyway . . . if someone wants to be different, that's OK providing it doesn't cause problems to other people. Respect for persons encompasses so much in terms of being aware of where people are.

She describes how her teaching strategies in experiential methods have developed from becoming aware of and utilizing role models when working alongside people in workshops, and also by reading to see what others have done. 'I've tried to think why it did or did not go well, and modify it accordingly'.

John Barnes describes one of the strengths of the course as the good relationship shared between the three people over the five years they have worked together: 'If we didn't work well together, it would affect the students.' Claire comments that the three share a common philosophy which Ruth believes is a long slow process of transmitting beliefs and values.

Figure 3.2 provides a summary of the three lecturers' professional backgrounds.

Teaching practice

Teaching practice occurs in blocks throughout the year. During each of the Autumn, Spring and Summer terms, three weeks is spent in a college of nursing. Additionally, a week's observation is spent in a college of higher education, and in the final few weeks of the course, the students spend one week in their own college.

The aim of the 11-week experience is to provide 'opportunities in which school, college teachers and course tutors share the role of preparing students for teaching' (The College, 1988). The first and third three-week experience usually occurs in the same hospital, and, if the student has not completed a recognized course, the middle three weeks is reserved for teaching in the practice setting.

	John Barnes	Claire Honeycutt	Ruth Copeman
Role	Overall Course tutor	Co-course tutor	Principal lecturer
Nursing qualifications Basic and advanced	RGN Sister tutor Diploma	SRN RSCN SCM Midwife teachers Diploma Diploma in nursing	RGN Clinical teacher Sister tutor Diploma
Professional qualifications	Diploma in Education MA (Ed) Curriculum Studies	BH First Class MA (Ed) Curriculum Studies	BA Hons 2:1 MSc Occupational Behaviour Pastoral Care and Counselling Course
Publications	Books	Journals	Journals
Teaching commitments on course	Educational psychology	Principles and practice of education	Human relationships

Figure 3.2   Profile of three staff members

Preparation for teaching practice

The first eight weeks of the academic year are organized to prepare students for their first placement. This includes input ranging from the preparation of lessons to teaching methods. Before this period ends, all students engage in peer group teaching sessions.

Claire stresses the importance of students finding their own style and describes this small piece of teaching as a 'practice run, a chance to put into practice the things they've been taught and have learned . . . mainly I want to boost confidence and get the newness over'.

The three lecturers all discussed the impact of themselves as role models. Claire says:

> 'We do practice what we preach. I hope they see a good standard of teaching, but realize no one is perfect, and there is not a paragon of virtue coming to see them.

Ruth elaborates:

> the way they're treated in class, the participative methods of teaching. There is encouragement for everybody to take part and do their bit and it develops them.

After the first placement the development of teaching skills in college occurs mainly through microteaching and students are also given opportunities to develop student-centred methods.

Figure 3.3 provides a breakdown of the teaching strategies used during five consecutive days teaching on the course.

Some factors affecting choice of teaching strategy

Research in general education provides an interesting comparison with the teaching strategies adopted by nurse teachers. Wragg (1972) used Flander's categories of analysis to demonstrate that most students had fixed patterns of teaching during teaching practice with only a small number varying their techniques. He suggests that the subject to be taught is the most important determinant of style, suggesting that styles can be linked to different subjects. Figures 3.4 to 3.8 demonstrate the strategies used by five students during the three placements (the students are the five who were watched during the non-participant observation, and their classification of methods during that session matched with mine). This demonstrates whether or not they broadened their repertoire of strategies as the experience progressed.

Fink (1976) found students became significantly more custodial towards pupils as the experience progressed, and were not as able to implement methods offered on the course as tutors would have liked.

	DAY 1	DAY 2	DAY 3	DAY 4	DAY 5
Subject	Term Evaluation	Teaching in Practice Settings	Educational Psychology	Human relationship skills	Educations
Topic		Review of Professional Practical Experience	Cognitive Styles	Communication in organizations	The management of change
Lecturer	John Barnes	Mary Hardcastle	John Barnes	Ruth Copeman	John Barnes/ Claire Honeycutt
Overall Method		Groupwork/ discussion	'Market stalls'	Experimental	Team teaching
Strategies	Nominal group techniques	Question and answer Groupwork Discussion	Advance organizers Timed experiments × 3 Exposition Discussion Post organizer	Brainstorm Exposition × 2 Questionnaire Role play	Advance organizers Small groupwork with Rating Scale Discussion × 2 JB Exposition CH Role play × 2 JB Question and answer × 2 CH Exposition × 2 JB Brainstorm CH Buzz group CH Post organizer
Subject	Education	Ethics	Therapeutic Communication	Tutorials	
Topic	Curriculum Planning				
Lecturer	Claire Honeycutt	Outside Speaker	Lydia Smith		
Overall Method	Modified Lecture/ Discussion	Lecture	Groupwork		
Strategies	Discussion × 2 Exposition × 2	Reading from notes Discussion	Exposition Question and answer		

Figure 3.3 Five days teaching strategies used at the college

Strategy	1	2	3
Exposition	5	5	5
Question and answer	5	2	1
Discussion		1	4
Groupwork	1	1	1
Brainstorm		1	
Demonstration	2	1	1
Supervised practice	2		
Guided study		2	
Quiz/questionnaire	1		
Video/film/tapeslide	2	1	1
Handouts		1	
Student feedback			1
Experimental exercises		1	
Role play	3	1	1
Advance organizers		1	
Springboard questions		1	

Figure 3.4 Summary of teaching strategies used by Paul on three placements

Strategy	1	2	3
Exposition	4	4	3
Question and answer	2	4	4
Discussion	1	1	
Groupwork	1	2	2
Brainstorm	1	1	
Buzz groups	1	1	1
Demonstration	1		
Quiz/questionnaire		1	
Video/film/tapeslide		1	
Handouts		1	1
Games	1		1
Experimental exercises		1	
Role play			1

Figure 3.5 Summary of teaching strategies used by Laura on three placements

Strategy	1	2	3
Exposition	1	1	2
Question and answer	2	6	4
Discussion	4	5	2
Groupwork	2	2	3
Brainstorm	2	2	
Buzz groups	1	1	1
Demonstration		1	1
Guided study		1	
Handouts	1		
Case study		1	
Role play		2	

Figure 3.6 Summary of teaching strategies used by Meg on three placements

Strategy	1	2	3
Exposition	8	6	7
Question and answer	11	7	7
Discussion	2	6	6
Groupwork	3	1	6
Brainstorm	3	3	4
Buzz groups	2	3	3
Quiz/questionnaire		1	
Video/film/tapeslide			1
Handouts		3	1
Case study			1
Games	3		
Experiential exercises	2		1
Advance organizer		2	2
Summary/answer		1	
Structured exercises			2
Springboard questions			1

Figure 3.7 Summary of strategies used by Tina on three placements

Strategy	1	2	3
Exposition	5		1
Question and answer	4		4
Discussion	3		1
Groupwork	2		1
Brainstorm		Clininal teaching practice	1
Demonstration	1		1
Quiz/questionnaire	1		2
Labelling diagram			1
Video/film/tapeslide	1		2
Dissecting animal organs			1
Role play	1		
Springboard questions			1

Figure 3.8 Summary of teaching strategies used by Kate on three placements

In addition to the information gained from the teaching diaries, the students identified many factors which contributed to influence their choice of teaching strategy. Laura reflected on the 'luck' of having small groups 'making it possible to attempt what had been taught'. Tina described how by the second placement,

> I got fired up to be a bit more bold and try different things. I got over my initial nerves and was only going there once so I could make a nit of myself. What happened was I went into 40–50 students in a lecture theatre, it killed all my lovely ideas of trying the bits we had been taught, people were lovely but the size of group was the criterion!

Pam felt her teaching was restricted by the number of teaching students on placement at the same time; the shortage of available teaching meant she did very little, leaving her with insufficient practice to meet her needs. In addition she said:

> I was able to do groupwork, but was restricted by subjects that had to be handled in a didacte way . . . I didn't teach the same group twice, didn't learn any names, I felt a total stranger, it inhibited factors I wanted to develop, I couldn't give my best.

She expressed disappointment at not being able to try experiential methods because of the subjects on offer to teach.

In contrast, Felicity chose the strategies that reflect how she likes to be taught 'high levels of interaction . . . experiential methods that fit in with my philosophy about teaching and nursing'.

Joyce felt more confident on the second placement:

> I was still nervous when I went into sessions, terrified really, because I'd chosen to use different methods. I was a bit straight on first T.P. . . . nothing too risky, but on the second one everything I did I tried to do differently, it was nerve wracking when it came to doing it.

She expressed concern over the hours she spend preparing classes, often over preparing, particularly for topics she was unfamiliar with, and felt she might have taken on too much teaching.

Anne commented: 'Your whole life changes for three weeks . . . I tried using what I'd been taught, interpersonal skills, methods of teaching'.

Carole reported that for one placement she received a letter with a list of subjects that she was to teach: 'I wouldn't normally touch them with a barge pole'. This made her feel she was there for the benefit of the school rather than to develop her own skills. She found a lack of freedom in choices of strategy:

> the tutors would say 'we want it done this way. It's always been done like that, use that video, discuss and finish. This is what we want'.

Paul also felt his choice of strategies was limited by the material offered to students:

> we did the sessions they didn't want . . . the A & P of sexuality they thought 'we'll foist it off on the students'.

Lucy coped in the following way:

> if I wasn't likely to teach a session again I refused to teach it on T.P. to make my preparation cost effective because of the hours spent on preparation you'll never use again!

Laura felt the school 'had a fixed idea of what I should do, when my ideas didn't match up, they said too much groupwork'. Meg reflected that a school's lack of interest in her meant 'I couldn't be bothered to prepare sessions'. In addition she found preparation at the school difficult as the office was unuseable due to noise. It seemed quite common for teacher students not to have a base in the school but to use desks vacated by tutors who were out for a day.

Lucy identified the lack of support as a factor which made her less adventurous; she felt reluctant to 'put myself in a situation where I'll fall flat on my face'.

Carole described one placement where her choice of strategy was 'opting for safety', except when team teaching with Lucy:

> the school didn't care what we did, they didn't even ask what we'd planned. the freedom was that no-one bothered to check.

In contrast, Felicity described the influence of a mentor who helped her to develop experiential teaching skills by team teaching with her over several sessions. She felt she was gradually 'eased' into a teaching role.

Meg felt that the mentor had potential to develop teaching strategies but

> people aren't prepared to sit in on your session, partly because they don't have the time, but they feel you want to find your feet.

Meg described how she asked if she could sit in and watch her mentor, but the request was refused.

> I tried the odd thing that I hadn't tried before. John says try things out, this is the time to do it, but there's not the facility for anybody to pick you up if it falls apart.
>
> I wanted someone around to say 'try this out, if it doesn't work it doesn't matter', but no-one was that free and easy, it was 'that's what's timetabled, this is what you cover', and I've been exposed to bad teachers and haven't suffered; the students won't be devastated if you do a session and the info doesn't get across as long as you admit it, .the school should create an atmosphere to allow it.

The size of the student group limited the strategies adopted. Tina reported the inhibiting effect of 'fifty in a lecture theatre'. Meg felt more confident with groups of eight in comparison to 50. 'I did try bits of role play, and that sort of thing', but she pursued the point that 'it was difficult to know if strategies had worked without a mentor present'. She added a final factor that influenced her teaching strategies:

> What I will take away from the course is the college staff as role models, then you can't do badly.

Boydell (1986) cautions that the end result of teaching practice is often the adoption of rigid, custodial impersonal teaching.

The effects of group size upon teaching and learning have been researched by De Cecco (1964). He found that despite student preferences for small groups there was no significant difference in the acquisition of information in groups varying from 15 to 67 members. Conversely Cantrell (1971) suggested that groups as large as 24 were both unpopular and inefficient, with maximum success achieved in groups of 12. Beard *et al.* (1976) support the latter view referring to the work of McKeachie (1966), suggesting that small groups are effective for retention, critical thinking and attitude change.

Clifton (1979) identifies a dilemma for teaching practice students, and questions whether they should follow the procedures of the 'supervising teacher' or the college lecturer. Lacey (1977) describes how cue conscious students adapt to social situations, but also questions whether the students should cue seek from the school placement or college.

Assessment of teaching

The students are assessed during each placement by a college lecturer, and by an internal assessor from the school of nursing. The visits from the college are rotated so that each student sees three different college assessors to give variety of feedback and to develop a broader student profile.

In the final term of the course lecturers submit a report on each student's performance. A board of assessors standardizes by sampling practical teaching assessments. If a candidate fails to satisfy the examiners, they are permitted to enter for reassessment on a maximum of two occasions within the three years following the first entry (The College, 1988).

John Barnes describes the aim of the visit as:

> to help students identify their teaching strengths, and areas where he or she needs to develop teaching skills through self-report and feedback.

He stresses that the focus of the assessment is formative, while confirming that assessment is important to maintain standards.

John encourages the students to experiment for the assessment and not just to 'play safe' to pass. He expects to see

> an overall modus operandi that they involve the group. If they miss opportunities for student involvement it's something I'd be hot to pick up, good questioning technique . . . I don't like scruffy overheads . . . giving it a go.

John describes the pleasure he gets from the visits, and misses the students when they're out of the college:

> they're usually quite glad to see me apart from the assessment angle . . . it gives me an opportunity to see them practising skills and gives feedback on what we do.

Figure 3.9 lists the behaviours that eight of the students felt merited reward in a teaching assessment. They felt the livelier the session the better, with a lot of activity and adventurous teaching, frequent changes of strategy,

• Rapport × 4	• Planning
• Flexibility × 2	• Novel ideas
• Manner	• Evaluation
• Student-centred	• Reinforcement
• Sound knowledge base	• Linked to psychology
• Creative AVAs	• Range of methods
• Lively presentation	• Humour
• Introduction	• Research
• Conclusion	• Andragogical principles
• Questioning skills	• Perfect OHPs
• Clinical application	

Figure 3.9   Eight students' predictions of assessment behaviour rewarded by John Barnes

minimum exposition and maximum experimentation; they thought John preferred to be involved in the session. They suggested that in an assessment situation he would be relaxed, professional, keen to put the students at ease, very enthusiastic but expecting a high standard. They predicted that in feedback he would be approachable, and would use the student's knowledge and contributions to link to future work. They also thought he would be uncritical and global in his views.

One of the sessions observed was Laura teaching seven new pupil nurses 'the prevention of pressure sores'. The experience began badly for me as I arrived, uncharacteristically, only three minutes before the session was due to begin and suspect that, of the trio, I was the one suffering with acute anxiety. John was quick to put me at ease. On the way to the classroom he put a reassuring arm around Laura. The students were sitting around desks arranged as a large table and Laura invited John to join the group. He quipped with the students 'I hope you can give me the answers' and there was lots of laughter. The students seemed happy and relaxed and there was teasing and banter between themselves, Laura and John, involving them in jokes, and humour throughout the session.

John checked that I was comfortable, took off his jacket and produced a pencil and sheet of A4 paper. The session adhered to the following format:

- question and answer
- exposition
- question and answer
- exposition
- buzz groups
- feedback
- handout
- exposition
- question and answer
- groupwork – case studies
- feedback.

During the session John appeared relaxed and pleased with events, he was smiling and warm, and his body posture was completely orientated to the student teacher. Occasionally he wrote a point down and seemed to think carefully about this, erasing one or two words and rewriting them, so he ended up with a list of ten points at the end of the session.

John entered into the relaxed informality of the classroom, nodding reinforcement to students' contributions, participating in buzz groups and groupwork, coaxing a rather shy student to explore ideas. Occasionally he referred to the lesson plan and frequently checked that I was all right. He appeared very relaxed. As the student teacher circulated around the students John teased her and encouraged her to relax, but fed back to her on the state of groupwork. He gently involved students in problem solving: 'yes, but he's got that tremor'. He prompted the students to use a flip chart and helped with spelling and writing. He smiled approvingly as Laura negotiated for an extra 10 minutes. At the end of the group feedback the students in his group spontaneously engaged in a congratulatory hand-shake at the standard of their work. On the way out of the classroom he said 'Well done! I think you're a lovely teacher'.

John allows for 30–60 minutes for feedback which is

> primarily about the process of teaching. If there were some aspects of content that I'm confident about I'd bring them up . . . and if there were conceptual problems I'd raise them . . . once a student confused emboli and thrombi as to which was static and which was mobile . . . but mainly process.

The feedback with Laura lasted 20 minutes. I was invited to join the interaction but sat in a corner of the office to observe. John asked Laura to reflect and evaluate, and asked for likes and dislikes. Laura was quick to point out that she left the OHP on for 10 minutes. John laughed and prompted for positive feedback, reinforcing each point and problem sol-ving with the student. 'What would you have got rid of?' He then worked through his list of ten points: 'seven good laudatory . . . three tiny points to consider'. On his page of notes the good points were indicated by the tick he placed next to them in order to prioritize his feedback. At the end of the session he invited comment from me and closed: 'excellent session, well done! . . . anything you want to ask me? . . . you've got all the skills for being a super teacher'. Laura: 'I wasn't nervous, I enjoyed it'.

The format was similar with the assessment of Tina, although he did not join the student group, John sat away from desk. Feedback to the student again lasted 15 minutes and consisted of ten points, three of which were areas to consider; he did suggest some experiential strategies instead of groupwork. Tina was so delighted that when showing me out of the school she gave me a huge hug and planted a kiss on my cheek, reinforcing for me the emotional quality of teaching and being assessed.

Ruth states her aim during the teaching practice visit:

> that the feedback I engage in will be a learning experience for them . . . trying to make the most of all the opportunities that offer themselves. If it seems as though a student has needs it's my job to do something about it. If the knowl-edge base in incorrect or if I can give them something to think about it's appropriate to do so; it's a matter of opportunities.

She acknowledged the 'high level of anxiety' that the assessment side of the visit contributed to: 'they know they're being judged and who likes that, a level of anxiety is always there'.

The students' predictions of the behaviour that Ruth would reward during an assessment are included as Figure 3.10. They felt she would expect the student teacher to be aware of the undercurrents of classroom mood, they felt she would 'work at every detail', would reward slow

- AVAs × 6
- Using students' ideas × 2
- Students at ease × 2
- Seating arrangements × 2
- Planning × 2
- Boardwork × 2
- Manner × 6
- Acceptance of students × 4
- Groupwork × 7
- Research-based × 2
- Timing × 2
- Content × 2
- Objectives
- Structure
- Clear speech
- Use of colour
- Writing in lower case
- Flexibility
- Questioning
- Clear instructions
- Links to future work
- Detailed background
- Varied methods
- Spelling
- Reinforcement
- Questioning

Figure 3.10 Eight students' predictions of assessment behaviour rewarded by Ruth Copeman

pacing of the lesson, allowing students the time to answer and think. They felt she would not penalize teacher-centred strategies.

The session I joined Ruth for was Meg teaching 'Sleep and Sleep Deprivation'. We travelled together to the hospital where Meg was waiting anxiously for us. In the 30 minutes before going into the session Meg expressed a great deal of distress about the placement and her experiences.

As we entered the large classroom the seven students stood and waited to be invited to sit down. It was a windy day and the noise in the classroom was considerable, not only from the weather but loud voices from the classroom next door. One of the students had a large starch rash above the uniform collar. The format of the session was as follows:

- warm up – small talk
- question and answer
- handout
- question and answer
- exposition
- buzz group
- question and answer

Ruth sat behind the L-shaped arrangement of students at a desk put there by Meg. She also had a sheet of A4 and a pencil and carefully followed the lesson plan, occasionally writing odd points on the sheet. She sat very quietly and remained still, but her face was animated and smiling and she seemed to enjoy the session immensely. Occasionally as I watched Meg teach, I noticed postures and traits which I felt were very characteristic of Ruth, slow speech, quiet voice, an open posture, long pauses after posing questions to allow students to think and extreme courtesy.

After the session Ruth offered Meg a recovery period and coffee was made, there was lots of laughter and humour as we drank this. The feedback was detailed lasting 75 minutes. Ruth invited Meg to reflect on how she felt about the session and invited her to work down the assessment form, self-assessing. Several times Meg asked for feedback, for example, on her questioning skills, she also frequently voiced difficulties about the placement. Ruth would listen sympathetically and was extremely supportive. Occasionally, she offered brief elaborations of the knowledge base, e.g. the causes of insomnia, the use of hypnotics. Meg continually returned to offloading some of her frustration. Ruth was gentle and supportive, continually reversing situations to encourage Meg to solve problems, but she continued to ask for a lot of reassurance. Ruth was sympathetic but her questions were probing; she asked for details of group preference for learning and asked searching questions about techniques: 'What did you think of . . . '. If Ruth commented on techniques, e.g. the use of coloured chalk or lower-case writing, she offered exposition and research findings to support her comment. The dialogue was punctuated by long silences which Meg broke. The feedback was a mixture of counselling, teaching and process.

On the journey back to London Ruth asked me for feedback, and seemed fascinated by the concept of a student modelling upon her. She normally allocates one hour for feedback after a session.

> I try to get most to put themselves on a continuum, occasionally if difficulties occur with a placement as a whole I might develop a counselling–guidance role, a bit about how to survive, a large part of me would like it to be a purely developmental role without assessment, but I think somebody has to say whether or not the person is suitable to be a teacher.

Claire Honeycutt interprets the intention of the teaching practice visit as

> to help with teaching, to give any tips, as much as possible to boost moral and confidence . . . we try to play down the assessment side, it's a joke, with the group we talk about visits . . . at the end of the day some assessment of whether they're competent or not to go and teach students has to be made, the quality of the teachers affects the quality of patient care.

Claire expresses a 'degree of discomfort' both with the use of classifying boxes on the assessment form and the ranking on the grids and would prefer to use an overall assessment of the person at the end of the course:

to have to give someone a borderline fail/pass is devastating to their confidence . . . . If someone is likely to be adversely affected by a bar on the grid at the extreme right-hand end I put an asterisk and a remark at the bottom of the page.

This tactic was evident in the assessment of Kate, which I joined, in which she asked for a student to demonstrate a skill without checking knowledge first. There was a potential for chaos. On the form under the heading 'Teacher–Learner Interactions' next to the statement 'responds appropriate to the differing needs and abilities of individual learners'. Claire placed an asterisk, and at the bottom of the form she commented: 'If you do get a student to demonstrate a procedure you need to watch them all the time'. She qualifies this tactic: 'the student needs to know if they've passed or not, but grades make the whole thing more nerve racking'.

It may discourage people from having a go and trying something different. There is a tendency to play safe. I think it's important for them not to feel like that, and try something new and see teaching as realistic with good and bad days. But there's pressure to pull out what's safe . . . I warm very much to people who pull out the stops and have a go. I say . . . 'if I come and you've never tried it before and its right for the group, do it!' . . . I like to see they've thought about what they've done.

She finds the visits pleasurable depending on how the students have done: 'if someone doesn't do very well I don't enjoy it, their confidence is shattered'.

The students felt that during an assessment Claire would be relaxed, professional and friendly, gentle and with a good rapport with them. They felt she would be accepting of their feelings but would reward flexibility, variety of method, experiential methods, high standards, sequencing and links with education. Figure 3.11 gives the list of behaviours that eight students suggested Claire would reward during a teaching assessment.

Claire and I travelled together to watch Paul teaching 'Control of Continence'. On arrival she requested a briefing of the format of the afternoon. Paul expressed concern 'over the stress of the assessment function'. He referred to an upsetting experience of an internal assessment which was very negative. Claire was reassuring and realistic about its significance; Paul explained he was trying new strategies for the session and he was visibly anxious.

The session was for 17 female students, several of whom were mature entrants. The classroom was large and airy with a skeleton and anatomical sections and models on shelves around the room. Claire and I sat in one corner and she rummaged in her large brief-case for the 'statutory' sheet of A4 and pencil.

- Manner × 6
- AVAs × 3
- Groupwork × 2
- Planning × 2
- Student participation
- Clear objectives
- Student contributions
- Sound knowledge base
- Positive reinforcement
- Research
- Questioning skills
- Theory to practice
- Handouts
- Humour
- Links to past learning
- Variety
- Sequencing

Figure 3.11 Eight students' predictions of assessment behaviour rewarded by Claire Honeycutt

The format of the lesson was as follows:

- springboard questions
- guided study
- handouts
- exposition
- question and answer
- exposition
- question and answer
- demonstration
- exposition
- question and answer.

The student teacher–student nurse rapport was evident as the sessions began:

> Student: 'Have you given up smoking?'
> Paul: 'No, I'm too stressed!'

Claire was laughing and enjoying the banter; one student commented on the nature of Paul's socks. Claire laughed loudly at this and continued to enjoy the repartee as the session progressed.

The demonstration was particularly memorable. The student had a large diagram of the pelvis, over which he held an inflated balloon, on which were stickers to demonstrate the bladder and its stretch receptors. There was considerable hilarity at the effort put into inflating the balloon, which Claire joined in, but the visual impact of the demonstration was high. Despite the presence of two 'college assessors' and lengthy interruption to the session, the students were able to ask quite intimate questions about stress incontinence which were handled skilfully.

During the session Claire wrote copious notes on her sheet of paper, occasionally scrubbling things out or asterisking items.

After the class had finished, tea was made and consumed before feedback during which Paul again discussed the stresses of teaching practice. The feedback was conducted in a small office. Claire began with 'How do you feel compared with the last assessment?'. Paul was able to identify strategies which pleased him and Claire probed continually: 'What was there about it that you liked?'. 'What did you do?'. Paul expressed fears of 'drying up' during a session and Claire offered several strategies to overcome this phenomenom.

Occasionally, Claire helped Paul through feedback by telling stories of her teaching strategies, usually hilariously funny. However, she was firm in her way of getting Paul to problem solve and develop his thinking. He admitted that he found self-evaluation difficult. Claire's approach was open and gentle and very caring. The feedback took 45 minutes, and was focused on teaching Paul how to develop his teaching strengths. Once this formal side was over, Paul again took 15 minutes to defuse over difficulties of the placement.

The journey back to London was memorable and reflects many of Claire's endearing qualities. Our discussion on the bus was so animated over the joys of teaching that we went several stops past the station and had to walk back! Once on the train, our debate continued but, having learned her lesson, Claire was searching for her station (several stops before mine) to the extent that, in the middle of a conversation, she jumped off the train, only to reveal the next day that it was a stop too soon!

John describes how assessing is standardized by talking with Claire and Ruth, and the fact that they share similar values. The three of them were part of a working group that redesigned the assessment form. John relates how he would prepare new staff members for their assessment role 'over coffee' talking through the form as a focus of discussion. He says that although he would share values he would ask them:

> to exercise independence. I would be quick to point out that there's no stereotype. New lecturers get quite anxious about it, they want to be credible.

Ruth describes the close degree of standardization that occurs as

> the hidden agenda could be a shared belief in the course philosophy. I suspect it's a long slow process of transmitting beliefs and values, while other assessors have themselves been students on the course.

Both John and Claire developed their techniques of assessing 'on the job'. Claire adds: 'informal discussion helps standardize, John and I discuss problems'. John elaborates upon how he develops self-assessment skills in the student by modelling the technique:

> and by formulating ground rules for peer group teaching in which I propose that feedback takes place in the following way: the students will have a few

minutes to reflect and then openly self-evaluate, the positive first and then bring up what we call points to consider, then the group would give feedback including myself.

Claire offers an example of how she models self-evaluation:

I might say at the end of a session I thought perhaps the groupwork went too long, and someone might say, 'yes it did!'. So they see teachers self-evaluating and it makes them feel it's respectable.

Ruth focuses feedback as 'individual idiosyncratic strengths' and how to develop them: 'I do sometimes give constructive criticism but lean heavily towards trying to get the person to see what they could do'.

A great deal has been written about the difficulties of assessing during teaching practice. Boydell (1986) identifies the complexity of the student teacher/supervisor, college lecturer triangle. He relates how the college lecturer is often reluctant to interfere with the 'master' (supervisor) and his apprentice. He believes that the supervisor is more influential than the college tutor. Additionally, he suggests that it is difficult for the college lecturer to amalgamate assessment, teaching and support in a visit. He found that students were often mistrusting of lecturers' assessments and suggests that it might interfere with the role of the school supervisor. This was evident in a small group of students:

more emphasis is placed on assessment than the lecturers care to admit . . . they're summatively assessed as well as being formative . . . there's a hidden agenda.

Stones and Morris (1972) consider that the college lecturers' power on teaching practice is minimal. They suggest that assessment generates anxiety in the students and limits experimentation so that they 'get it right' on the day. They note that assessment is often an idiosyncrasy of a particular college, unstandardized and unsystematic. Stones and Morris contend that the assessment role weakens the function of the advisor and this may also be true of the school supervisor in a dual role.

Becher (1982) indicates that assessment feedback correlates positively with high student achievement while Walker (1981) argues that formal evaluation is a myth used to ensure and monitor conformity. He claims that perception ensures that an assessor sees what the teacher ought to be doing, so that the events of a session may be the constructs of an assessor's expectations. He argues for a negotiated feedback which depends upon the student's needs, and describes the use of a standardized form.

Flanders' ten categories of interaction analysis were used by Wragg (1971) to study the effects of systematic and unsystematic feedback upon students' teaching. He found that feedback reduces the amounts of straight lecturing and increases the amount of pupil interaction in a lesson. He argues that feedback is a powerful means of influencing behaviour and increasing competence. Wragg (1982) also highlights the difficult and subjective nature of assessing teaching. He refers to a study in which 35 tutors were asked to rate taped teaching sessions, grades awarded ranged from B+ to D for the same scenario. Foy (1969) reports on one teacher rated for 44 characteristics on two occasions separated by 30 months. The results correlated significantly (0.71). Gage (1978) conversely demonstrates that assessment hardly influences a student's teaching.

Fontana (1972) questions what assessors are looking for in teaching practice. Follow-up studies demonstrate that the final teaching mark is of questionable value in predicting success. He asks what measurable qualities in a student's performance make for good teaching marks. He says crucial issues revolve around the value systems involved in subjective judgements and the extent to which college supervisors agree about what to assess.

The students had a great deal to say about their experiences of assessment. Meg described the sleepless nights before assessments but added that she was left with a 'positive feeling' once they were over. She described how she 'tailored' her teaching to the assessor:

> with John I felt if there was not a lot of interaction I would be penalized, so the way round it was to split them into groups. John like it, the students liked it, it was effective . . . with Ruth it didn't matter so much, things could be less explicit.

She described her aim in an assessment as 'getting through without a disaster, it's very stressful, it's important, and it's a hassle, the students are unknown and so much rides on it'. Meg felt the college assessment could be taken seriously. She described how college assessors expect to see theory put into practice: 'their feedback is the most valuable thing on TP'.

Tina said of the college assessment: 'it's the only time we get truly assessed as individuals, you truly know what you're doing, it's for you not the group'.

Felicity felt the college assessment 'gives freedom to develop in a way that's appropriate for individuals'.

Anne described the college lecturers as supportive and guiding, 'although the official reason is minimized it's threatening, the lectures are most helpful'.

Joyce revealed the high levels of anxiety she experienced on teaching practice: 'I lost so much weight'. She related how when preparing for an assessment 'everything has to be perfect. I spent two hours preparing one OHP'.

Lucy felt her assessment with Ruth:

> was wonderful, what I got out of it was tremendous, she's so skilled that not only did I feel good for myself, I sussed her out and thought how did she do that? So I can use it as an assessment tool, not once did she comment, she got me to identify strengths and weaknesses in such a way that it wasn't detrimental it was constructive . . . it didn't feel like an assessment.

Conclusion

Traditionally the researcher does not draw conclusions from a case study, but leaves the reader to extract their own meaning from the findings. However, I am going to mention a few of the more overt personal implications of this work. First, the study clearly demonstrated to me the emotional nature both of teaching and researching. Both aspects of an educator's role appear fragile and susceptible to many influences.

Curriculum developers have to consider how to maximize the advantages of teaching practice, while planning strategies to overcome the limitations of such an experience.

The sample for this study is small, and this chapter represents about one-third of the complete project. This makes the findings difficult to generalize from.

Most of the literature used to create concepts and underpin the study came from general education, from mature pieces of work which have been published in the last decade. It is difficult to assess what the differences are between a nurse teacher's role and those teachers working in the general education sector.

In attempting to answer questions, new questions emerged to tease! While I would not wish to restrict the case study worker I would suggest that the student conforming to a word limit finds some way of pacing their research, perhaps by answering one question at a time, to a time scale. I tended to collect data for different themes simultaneously and at times was swamped with information, some of which I could not use.

Finally, the insights I gained from this study have had an enormous impact upon the curriculum and upon my personal understanding of the process of being a teaching student on the courses at the college. The findings from this section of the study presented to the course curriculum development group had the following impact. First, and most significantly, students no longer slot into allocated number of teaching practice places. Instead, students receive guidance on what to look for in a practice placement and make their own arrangements. This has greatly reduced the potential for a person/environment mismatch and although it still does occur it is unusual.

Secondly, course members are certainly encouraged to reflect on their placement experiences both through a personal medium and during regular planned sessions facilitated by a lecturer in the college.

Thirdly, although the number of summative teaching practices has remained, students are required to undertake a minimum of four formative assessments during their placements, which should help them develop personal awareness of their teaching style, both strengths and areas to develop. This has been positively evaluated by course members and they suggest that this activity strengthens the relationship between the student and supervisor.

The student teacher assessment form has been redesigned and requires a series of statements to be made but not graded. An overall pass/fail decision is then made.

Students are encouraged to consider carefully the amount of teaching that they take on board. The college now suggests that 2–3 hours per 5 days is more than enough if learning is to take place.

Finally, instead of a college lecturer visiting a student on three occasions, two of the summative assessments have been developed to the supervisor. This also seems to have significantly reduced the stress associated with assessment although I suspect that the status of one visit has been inflated in the students' minds to a major event.

The following chapters focus on varying aspects of and approaches to research, with accounts of difficulties and suggestions that can help the novice researcher make informed choices and a few shortcuts.

References

Adelman C (Ed.) (1981) *Uttering Muttering*. Grant McIntyre, London.

Beard R *et al.* (1976) *Research into Teaching Methods in Higher Education Mainly in British Universities*, 3rd edn. Penguin, Middx.

Becher R M (1982) The relationship of field placement characteristics and students potential field performance abilities to clinical experience performance ratings. *Journal of Teacher Education* XXXIII (2), 24–30.

Bennett N (1976) *Teaching Styles and Pupil Progress*. Open Books, London.

Boydell D (1986) Issues in teaching practice supervision research: a review of the literature. *Teaching and Teacher Education* 2 (2), 112–25.

Burgess R G (1984) *In the Field: An Introduction to Field Research*. Allan & Unwin, London.

Cantrell E G (1971) Thirty lectures. *British Journal of Medical Education* 5 (4), 300–19.

De Cecco P (1964) Class size and coordinated instruction. *British Journal of Eduational Psychology* 34 (1), 65–74.

Clifton R A (1979) Practice teaching: survival in a marginal situation. *Canadian Journal of Education* 4 (3), 60–74.

Cohen L and Manion L (1985) *Research Methods in Education*, 2nd edn. Croom Helm, London.

The College (1988) *Curriculum Document*. Internal publication.

Fink C H (1976) *Social Studies Student Teachers What do They Really Learn?* Paper presented at the Annual Meeting of the National Council for the Social Studies, Washington DC Nov. 4–7.

Fontana D (1972) What do we mean by a good teacher? In Chanan D (Ed.) *Research Forum on Teacher Education*. NFER, Windsor.

Foy J M (1969) A note on lecturer evaluation by students. *Universities Quarterly* 23 (3), 42–88.

Gage N L (1978) *The Scientific Basis of the Art of Teaching.* Teachers College Press, New York.

Lacey C (1977) *The Socialisation of Teachers.* Methuen, London.

Lofland J (1971) *Analysing Social Settings.* Wadsworth, California.

McKeachie W J (1966) Research in teaching the gap between theory and practice. In *Improving College Teaching.* American Council on Education, Washington.

Nisbett J and Watt J (1978) *Case Study.* T.C.R. Rediguide, University of Aberdeen.

Parlett M and Hamilton D (1972) Evaluation as illumination: a new approach to the study of innovatory programmes. In *Occasional Paper* 9. Centre for Research in the Educational Studies, University of Edinburgh.

Patton M D (1980) *Qualitative Evaluation Methods.* Sage, London.

Pollard A (1984) Opportunities and difficulties of a teacher – Ethnographer: a personal account. In Burgess R G (1985) *The Research Process in Educational Settings: Ten Case Studies.* Falmer Press, Lewes.

Pring P (1984) Confidentiality and the right to know. In Adelman C (Ed.) *The Politics and Ethics of Evaluation.* Croom Helm, London.

Royal College of Nursing of the United Kingdom (1977) *Ethics Related to Research in Nursing.* RCN, London.

Ruddock J (1985) The improvement of the art of teaching through research. *Cambridge Journal of Education* 15 (3), 123–7.

Scott S (1985) Working through the contradictions in researching postgraduate education. In Burgess R G (Ed.) *The Research Process in Educational Settings: Ten Case Studies.* Falmer Press, Lewes.

Simons M (1981) Conversation Piece. In Adelman C (Ed.) *Uttering Muttering.* Grant McIntyre, London.

Stenhouse L (1984) A note on case study and educational practice. In Burgess R G (Ed.) *Field Methods in the Study of Education.* Falmer Press, Lewes.

Stenhouse L (1975) *An Introduction to Curriculum Development and Research.* Heinemann, London.

Stones E and Morris S (1972) *Teaching Practice Problems and Perspectives.* Methuen, London.

Treece W and Treece J (1982) *Elements of Research in Nursing.* Mosby, St Louis.

Walker R T (1981) Myths in student teacher evaluation. *English Education* 13 (1), 10–16.

Walker R (1980) The conduct of educational case studies. In Dockrell W B and Hamilton D (Eds) *Rethinking Educational Research.* Princeton Book Co., New Jersey.

Woods P (1985) Ethnography and theory construction in educational research. In Burgess R G (Ed.) *The Research Process in Educational Settings: Ten Case Studies.* Falmer Press, Lewes.

Wragg E C (1971) The influence of feedback on teachers' performance. *Educational Research* June, 218–21.

Wragg E C (1972) An analysis of the verbal interaction between graduate student teachers and children. Unpublished PhD thesis, Exeter University.

Wragg E C (1982) *A Review of Research in Teacher Education.* NFER – Nelson, London.

4

Fostering critical thinking in nurse education: the development of a measurement tool

Marion Allison

'(There) is one characteristic of the good research problem – that it be of interest to the researcher.' (Fox, 1982, p. 80)

This chapter provided in depth analysis of critical thinking as a bonus. It also:

- *maps the development of a research problem through a literature review;*
- *clearly demonstrates an analytical writing style which we all strive for. This is difficult to describe but recognizable when you read it;*
- *plots the development of a research tool;*
- *demonstrates how to use and report on a pilot study;*
- *discusses issues of reliability and validity.*

Introduction

This chapter focuses on the development of a tool to identify and measure the teaching strategies used by teachers in the classroom to promote the development of critical thinking skills in pre-registration nursing students.

The publication of Project 2000 (UKCC, 1986) outlined a radical new framework for the organization and delivery of pre-registration nursing education. In common with colleagues working in this field of nurse education, I recognized the profound implications it would have on all aspects of my role, from curriculum planning to evaluating the effectiveness with which the new programme would achieve intended outcomes.

As I became familiar with the document and its proposals, I began to question my current teaching practices and my work with nursing students in the classroom setting. The report requires the nurse practitioner to be a thinking person with analytical skills and states that programmes of initial preparation should be at such a level that they enable students to develop the ability to think analytically and flexibly. I recognized that, if these requirements were to be met, it was important to have an accurate perception of the nature of critical thinking and to determine whether teachers are using appropriate teaching strategies to promote the development of critical thinking skills. The following discussion explains the nature of the concept of critical thinking, explores how critical thinking can be fostered in nursing students and outlines the process through which a data collection tool was devised which assesses whether students are provided with opportunities in basic nurse education programmes to use and develop specific critical thinking abilities. This tool is multipurpose: it also provides a framework to enable teaching to be structured so that the development of critical thinking is deliberately fostered, and serves as a method of self-evaluation.

Initial review of the literature

My initial intention in searching the published literature was to increase my understanding of the concept and to gain an overview of current knowledge of critical thinking in nurse education. Reading at this stage consisted of both conceptual and research-based literature (Fox, 1982).

During this preliminary review I learned that concern for the development of higher order thinking skills was not restricted to nursing education in the United Kingdom. In the United States for several years, articles in professional journals had discussed effective strategies for teaching students how to think and process information accurately and published research reports documented the investigation and measurement of critical thinking ability in nursing students and qualified nurses: both provided evidence of a growing interest in the role of critical thinking in nursing and academic performance.

Since 1989, the development of higher order thinking skills has been viewed as an essential component of nurse education in the United States. As part of the process for the accreditation of baccalaureate programmes, the National League for Nurses requires that nursing schools provide evidence that planned curricula promote critical thinking, decision making and independent judgement (NLN, 1989).

Similar concerns were evident in the field of general education. As a member of the 'teaching for thinking' movement, Paul (1984) believed that 'without the ability to think, without the ability to reason, students are intellectually, emotionally, and morally incomplete' (p. 4). Paul (1987) differentiated educated people from those who had been trained by particular criteria: 'they achieve a grasp of critical principles and an ability and passion to choose, organise and shape their own ideas and living beliefs by means of them' (p. 145).

Nickerson (1987) answered the question 'why teach thinking' by listing the consequences of failure to do so:

> blindly following authority, acting without thought for the consequences of our actions, having our opinions moulded and our behaviour shaped by illogical arguments . . . believing the future will be what it will be and taking no steps to make it what it could be, and failing to make any effort to see things from other people's points of view. (p. 36)

Thinking is generally assumed to be a cognitive process, or mental act by which knowledge is acquired (Preseissen, 1985). It is accepted that thinking skills are not of a single kind, and they are not all equal (Sternberg, 1987). Beyer (1985a) distinguished between lower skills and complex multiprocess thinking strategies, a stance consistent with that of others. Four different complex thinking processes or 'macro-process strategies', problem solving, decision making, critical thinking and creative thinking, which require the use of multiple essential basic thinking skills, have been proposed (Cohen, 1971). The basic cognitive skills involved in these macro-process strategies were analysed by Beyer (1985a), who concluded that there was often overlap in the reasoning tasks required to effectively undertake them.

Ennis (1987) has defined critical thinking as reasonable, reflective thinking that is focused on deciding what to believe or do and as a purposeful mental activity that helps to formulate or solve problems, make decisions, or fulfil a desire to understand (Walters, 1986). The concept of critical thinking can be viewed as a framework into which the reasoning skills required for the previously listed complex thinking processes can be incorporated. The development of critical thinking abilities would appear to be of value for professional nurses and constitute an important part of education for clinical nursing practice. Their need has been succinctly stated by Malek (1986):

> As members of a profession in which situations change rapidly, nurses cannot depend upon routine behaviour, procedure manuals or traditions to guide clinical judgement and decision making. They must develop the ability to make guided decisions drawn from sound rational bases. (p. 20)

The exercise of well-developed thinking skills is, therefore, essential if nurses are to be safe, competent and skilful. Pardue (1987) noted that the cognitive processes required to use and implement the nursing process were the same as those defined for critical thinking ability; through linking theory and practice, the nursing process is an instrument which can promote and enhance critical thinking.

Opinion is still divided about whether critical thinking is an innate ability or a system of learned and taught skills (Walters, 1986), although most experts would agree that students can be taught to think more effectively (Nickerson, 1987). Disagreement exists about whether the teaching of thinking should be the focus of special exercises, tests and programmes separate from the curriculum, or integrated into the delivery of existing curricula (Sternberg, 1987). There is sufficient evidence to suggest that critical thinking skills learned in isolation are not transferred to other areas (Glatthorn and Baron, 1985). The separatist approach has been criticized by McPeck (1981) who stated that:

> purporting to teach critical thinking in the abstract, in isolation from specific fields or problem areas, is muddled nonsense; thinking of any kind is always 'thinking about X'. Critical thinking cannot be a distinct subject. (p. 13)

Thus critical thinking cannot be separated from a specific context, and is always tied to distinct areas of expertise and knowledge. This has implications for nurse educators for, if nurse practitioners of the future are to think critically about their professional practice, their critical thinking skills will have to be developed within a conceptual understanding of nursing. Exposure to, and practice of, appropriate teaching and learning strategies for the cultivation of effective critical thinking have to be integrated into this nursing context. It becomes the nurse teacher's responsibility in basic nursing education courses to facilitate the acquisition of critical thinking skills over time in classroom and clinical situations so that the student's professional nursing practice becomes informed and guided by a proclivity for critical thinking.

Interest in improving critical thinking skills suggests the need to evaluate those skills (Baron, 1987). The Cornell Critical Thinking Tests (Ennis and Millman, 1985) and the Watson Glaser Critical Thinking Appraisal Test (Watson and Glaser, 1980) are the two most widely used critical thinking tests, both of which employ a multiple choice format. Their approach is to evaluate thinking skills outside the context of course content; so far, only one topic-specific critical thinking test has been reported in the literature (Kneedler, 1985), a major part of which also consists of multiple choice questions. Previous studies of critical thinking ability in a nursing context provide some information on the impact of the nursing curriculum on the development of critical thinking skills and on differences in critical thinking among nurses with different levels of preparation.

Frederickson (1979) conducted a pilot study on 14 volunteer baccalaureate students, measuring changes in critical thinking ability over time using the Watson Glaser Critical Thinking Appraisal (WGCTA) Test, and concluded that their abilities for critical thinking improved over the duration of the course. In 1987, Gross, Takazawa and Rose used an accessible sample of 71 associate and baccalaureate degree students to investigate differences in critical thinking abilities at the commencement and completion of their programmes. Of the students who completed the course, there was a significant improvement in critical thinking abilities in both groups when measured by the WGCTA test. An additional finding was that students who dropped out of the associate degree course had higher WGCTA scores on entry than those who went on to complete both programmes. The researchers suggested that these students could possibly not have been challenged by this course, although the students' reasons for leaving were not investigated to provide support for this assertion. It was concluded that nursing education had improved critical thinking in those students who completed the programmes.

In contrast, Sullivan (1987) used the WGCTA test on 46 volunteer baccalaureate students to measure critical thinking ability at the beginning of the first year and at the end of their last semester. The mean score obtained by students on both tests was consistent at 57 out of a possible total score of 80. Bauwens and Gerhard (1987) conducted a similar study on 53 baccalaureate students and also found no change in the WGCTA scores in their sample between the first and last semesters.

Differences in critical thinking abilities in a sample of 121 nurses with different levels of preparation, from masters to associate degree students were investigated by Pardue (1987). She found that scores on the WGCTA test increased with higher levels of preparation, from 52 in associate degree nurses to 64 in masters prepared nurses, with diploma and baccalaureate nurses occupying intermediate positions.

The only study purporting to explore critical evaluation skills actually used by student nurses was conducted by Keeley, Browne and Kreutzer in 1982. A small sample of nursing students was asked to write an essay in which they critically evaluated a written passage. It is not clear what specific instructions they were given. The study findings suggested that only half the students could identify examples of ambiguity, illogical flow, or misuse of data within the passage.

The majority of these studies focused on the measurement of critical thinking abilities using one specific test, the WGCTA. The results presented were inconclusive; some students increased their initial scores when tested again at the end of nursing programmes while for others, the results were unchanged.

The WGCTA is a widely available standardized test for measuring critical thinking ability. However, the reliability of the test has been called into question by McPeck (1981), who claimed that within the test and its instructions there are inconsistencies which actually preclude the use of critical thinking, and further suggested that it is uncertain whether critical thinking as a unique set of skills is actually being tested. The skills tested differ considerably from those included in Ennis and Millman's (1985) Cornell Tests of Critical Thinking, not only in terms of the specific skills measured, but in the nature and structure of these tests as a whole. It has been pointed out that whether an individual is proficient in critical thinking may depend on whose test or inventory of critical thinking is used as a standard measurement (Beyer, 1985a). Since neither the Cornell nor the WGCTA tests are content specific, it is unknown if students who achieved high scores on such a test thought critically about their nursing knowledge or clinical work. Since our aim as educators is to produce nurses who do possess the ability to think critically about their nursing practice it seems imperative that a means is developed by which to assess these abilities in nursing and to determine the influence of the education process in their development.

The initial review was invaluable in clarifying my thoughts, developing my understanding of current knowledge of critical thinking in nursing and identifying areas which required further investigation. There was an undisputed need for future nurse practitioners to develop the ability to think analytically and flexibly and for basic nurse education programmes to foster effective critical thinking, since this concept incorporates reasoning skills required in other complex thinking processes. It was widely accepted that students can be taught to think more effectively, but critical thinking is context specific so such teaching has to be integrated into nursing courses in such a way that students develop a propensity for critical thinking and become effective critical thinkers in their clinical practice.

Previous studies in this area were limited in scope and inconclusive in determining whether nursing courses have a positive effect on the development of critical thinking skills; the only test used so far has been criticized as a valid measure of critical thinking ability. There was no research based knowledge about the concept of critical thinking in United Kingdom nursing programmes and no tool available with which to measure the critical thinking abilities nursing students need to acquire. It is not known whether teachers use strategies which foster critical thinking in pre-registration education courses.

I considered that there was little value in measuring differences in nursing students' critical thinking abilities unless the skills embodied within the concept of critical thinking were clearly identified and a method devised for assessing whether students are provided with opportunities in basic nursing education programmes to use and develop those specific abilities. Identification of these specific critical thinking skills and abilities can provide a conceptual framework from which to develop a tool to monitor whether teachers use appropriate teaching strategies to promote the development of particular skills. This tool will make it possible to ascertain whether nurse education programmes do contribute to the development of critical thinking; furthermore, I considered that the information gained could provide a foundation for further study to determine whether teachers have an accurate perception of critical thinking and adequate preparation for the promotion of critical thinking in nurse education. Knowledge of whether critical thinking is encouraged in nursing students will provide valuable information on the current situation in nurse education and help to determine whether action needs to be taken to ensure that critical thinking opportunities are incorporated into nurse education programmes. My purpose became clearer and more defined as I critically reviewed the available literature, and it was my intention to develop a Critical Thinking Teaching Strategies Analysis (CTTSA) tool which could measure the strategies used by nurse teachers to foster the development of critical thinking skills in students undertaking basic nurse education programmes.

The following sections of the chapter discuss the literature review undertaken in detail, as this published work in the field of critical thinking provided the theoretical foundation from which the measurement tool was devised.

Critical thinking

There has been considerable discussion on the meaning of the concept of critical thinking. Although some researchers have equated critical thinking with problem solving, decision making and creative thinking (Fraenkel, 1980), most would agree that these are more accurately described as closely related cognitive skills (Cohen, 1971) and that critical thinking operates in each of these complex thinking processes. Beyer (1985a) suggests that imprecise definitions which confuse critical thinking with other thinking skills fail to distinguish its unique features; he maintains that a consensus description about the nature of critical thinking is essential if the goal of improving student competency is to be attained. Although this has not yet been achieved it is possible to find areas of commonality within the literature about the fundamental nature of critical thinking and thus identify key critical thinking skills.

In 1962, Ennis produced a thorough analysis of critical thinking, based on an extensive search of psychological, philosophical and educational research. He has since refined his interpretation to produce a definition of critical thinking as 'reasonable reflective thinking that is focussed on deciding what to believe or do' (Ennis, 1987, p. 10). From Ennis' perspective, critical thinking is a personal activity which includes higher order thinking skills such as those listed in Bloom's (1956) taxonomy of analysis, synthesis and evaluation. In his later work he also claims that critical thinking involves creative elements which permit the production of ideas and alternatives and provides examples of these which include formulating hypotheses, asking questions, viewing a problem in different ways, suggesting possible solutions and devising plans for investigation. Kurfiss (1988) stated that critical thinking is 'an investigation whose purpose is to explore a situation, phenomenon, question or problem to arrive at a hypothesis or conclusion about it that integrates all available information and that therefore can be convincingly justified' (p. 2).

From these definitions it can be established that critical thinking is a process which involves careful, persistant and objective analysis of knowledge, beliefs, or situations to judge their validity or worth. The accepted outcome of critical thinking is therefore to reach a conclusion and to offer justification in support of it. Ennis (1987) goes on to assert that critical thinking should form the basis for subsequent action; this belief is consistent with Russell's (1956) earlier work (cited by Beyer, 1985a); Russell thought that the process of critical thinking ends with the expression of judgements in subsequent action.

Critical thinking skills

Critical thinking has been described as consisting of two components: a frame of mind and a number of specific mental operations (Beyer, 1985a). He cites Fraser and West's (1961) work to illustrate the components of this disposition, in which they suggested that it involved an alertness to the need to evaluate information, a willingness to test opinions and a desire to consider all viewpoints. Ennis (1987) accepts this view; in addition, he includes taking into account the total situation, being open-minded, taking a position and changing it when the evidence and reasons are sufficient to do so, and dealing in an orderly manner with parts of a complex whole in his own list of dispositions. McPeck (1981) described critical thinking as the propensity and skill to engage in an activity with reflective scepticism. For McPeck (1981) scepticism, or the suspension of assent, directed towards a given statement, established norm, or mode of doing things, should be productive of a more satisfactory solution, or insight into, the problem at hand. It includes the consideration of alternative hypotheses and possibilities and ensures that, although the student may ultimately arrive at acceptance, he does not take truth for granted. This highlights a fundamental aspect of critical thinking – the ability to engage in reflection and deliberation, to weigh the evidence, and only then to reach a tentative conclusion (Glatthorn and Baron, 1985). As a mental activity, critical thinking is not a single act such as recall, and as a process can be differentiated from problem solving which consists of a sequential series of discrete cognitive strategies; critical thinking is a collection of separate skills which all incorporate elements of analysis and evaluation (Beyer, 1985a). It is possible to identify key critical thinking skills from the published literature of theorists and educational researchers.

The work of Morse and McCune, first published in 1940, drew together published ideas and research on the nature of critical thinking and was used as a resource for later work, such as that of Fraser and West (1961), who described six critical thinking skills: determining the relevance of material, evaluating the reliability of authors, differentiating between fact and opinion, evaluating assumptions, checking the accuracy of data and detecting inconsistencies.

Brown and Cook (1971) carried on the work of Morse and McCune (1965). The six skills they identified were consistent with those of previous authors, but they also listed four skills of critical mindedness: refraining from jumping to conclusions, retaining an open mind, evaluating given sources of information, and analysing related parts of a problem. The first two seem to be dispositions, or evidence of a certain frame of mind, which fit into the dimension of critical thinking previously discussed, but the last two are cited as critical thinking skills or abilities by other authors (Watson and Glaser, 1980; Ennis, 1987) so would appear to be more appropriately categorized in this way. Hudgins (1977) conducted a research based literature review and produced a list of specific critical thinking skills which consisted of finding information, detecting bias – especially in terms of unreliability and overgeneralizing, evaluating a line of reasoning, weighing evidence, finding unstated assumptions, and identifying both ambiguous and equivocal statements. Other early work published by Dressel and Mayhew in 1954 was used by Watson and Glaser (1980) as the basis for the instrument they developed for their critical thinking test, which encompassed five skills: determining the probable accuracy of an inference, including identifying the inference itself, recognizing assumptions, deducing conclusions, interpreting information and evaluating the strength of an argument in terms of its relevance and importance to a question. Finally, Ennis' (1987) taxonomy of critical thinking dispositions and abilities represented the culmination of his work on this concept over 25 years, and is the most fully developed framework, being divided into four basic areas labelled clarification, basis, inference and interaction, into which critical thinking skills are categorized.

Clarification is subdivided into an elementary level which includes analysing arguments, the ability to focus on a question, identifying a problem or hypothesis and asking appropriate clarifying questions. Advanced clarification involves defining terms and identifying assumptions; support for one's inferences lies within the area of basis and includes judging the credibility of a source and observing and judging observation reports; inference involves deduction, induction and making value judgements. Ennis (1987) points out that the above abilities focus on acquiring reasonable beliefs, and are valuable for the role they play in reaching reasonable decisions about what to do. However, he includes the elements of the process of problem solving as a way of organizing the approach to deciding on an action, as a separate aspect of critical thinking ability. Within his classification, the final category is interaction (or strategy and tactics), and it is here that the practical application or 'action' of the previous three areas of critical thinking takes place. He goes into further detail, by specifying the attributes of each type of skill listed. It is his contention that the actual practice of critical thinking requires the combination of these abilities and their employment in conjunction with critical thinking dispositions and knowledge of the subject.

Despite some diversity among the skills labelled as critical thinking, a well substantiated consensus about the nature of critical thinking and its key cognitive operations can be derived from the synthesis of expert views in the field of critical thinking and this formed the basis of seminal work by Beyer (1985a), who compiled a list of the 10 key skills that reflect this

1. Distinguishing between verifiable facts and value claims
2. Determining the reliability of a source
3. Determining the factual accuracy of a statement
4. Distinguishing relevant from irrelevant information, claims or reasons
5. Detecting bias
6. Identifying unstated assumptions
7. Identifying ambiguous or equivocal claims or arguments
8. Recognizing logical inconsistencies or fallacies in a line of reasoning
9. Distinguishing between warranted and unwarranted claims.
10. Determining the strength of an argument

Figure 4.1   Ten key critical thinking skills identified by Beyer (1985a)

consensus (Figure 4.1). Although, as previously described, other individuals have proposed additional critical thinking skills, the list contains
those most commonly advanced and such refinements are required if we
are to be clear about what constitutes critical thinking. An essential aspect
of critical thinking is the suspension of assent until, through reflection,
deliberation and the analysis of evidence and alternatives, a reasonable
conclusion or judgement is reached. The 10 skills listed are essential
elements of this process.

Critical thinking in the curriculum

Most researchers agree that students do not acquire good thinking skills as
a consequence of studying certain subjects, assimilating the products of
someone else's thinking, or being asked to think about a subject or topic
(McPeck, 1981). This point has been emphasized by Glaser (1985) who
stated:

> a student does not tend 'naturally' to develop a general disposition to consider
> thoughtfully the subjects and problems that come within the range of his or her
> experience; nor is he or she likely to acquire knowledge of the methods of
> logical inquiry and reasoning and skill in applying these methods, simply as a
> result of having studied this subject or that. There is little evidence that stu-
> dents acquire skill in critical thinking as a by product of the study of any given
> subject. (p. 27)

The direct teaching of critical thinking as a separate skill has been advocated (Beyer, 1985b; Wright, 1985), but the effectiveness of such programmes has been questioned (Paul, 1987; Perkins, 1987). McPeck (1981)
asserts that reasoning is the judicious use of scepticism applied to the
norms and standards of the field under consideration and that thinking
cannot be divorced from the skills that make the field of activity what it is –
'insofar as critical thinking involves knowledge and skill, a critical thinker
in area X might not be a critical thinker in area Y' (McPeck, 1981, p. 13).
The ability to transfer critical thinking skills cannot be assumed. Following

a review of available evidence in this area, Grant (1988) concluded that the best approach in teaching critical thinking is within the disciplinary areas of the curriculum. Her opinion is supported by Shulman (1974) who stated:

> it is abundantly clear that no amount of general intellectual skill or mastery over cognitive strategies will overcome lacks in content knowledge. It seems reasonable to assume that a fairly complex set of knowledge by process inter-actions is involved in the construct we call clinical competence. (p. 325)

From a nursing education perspective, Miller and Malcolm (1990) argue that critical thinking is dependent upon a knowledge base on which argu-ments can be built and also that the discipline of nursing would be greatly assisted if teachers recognize that critical thinking is required in the appli-cation of existing knowledge but that it is also imperative for developing the knowledge base of the discipline: 'faculty need to convey to students that, indeed, there is a paradigm of nursing science being developed and that, as professionals, they can and should contribute to that science through inquiry and critical thinking' (p. 71). If this is to be achieved, opportunities for developing critical thinking need to be embedded within nurse education programmes; efforts to instil critical thinking dispositions and abilities should be an intrinsic aspect of the nursing course and applied within the context of teaching and learning about the field of nursing studies.

Teaching critical thinking

Within the literature, many methods have been suggested through which teachers can promote critical thinking in nursing students. Schank (1990) listed several strategies which included using simulation, individually or in groups, which required written or verbal evaluation of outcomes, indepen-dent projects such as research critiquing, care plan development, or speci-fically designed teaching materials as methods for developing skills of enquiry and analysis. She also suggest using the case incident to help students practise reflective thinking skills in the process of decision making.

> Students study the incident to find out what is going on, to identify what more needs to be known, to obtain and organise the needed information and to identify the real issue. They then formulate a decision with concomitant rationale and identify what was learned in the broader context from this incident for future reference. (Schank, 1990, p. 88)

She further demonstrated how techniques used in general education could be effectively adapted by nurse teachers, using Rhoades and Rhoades' (1985) ideas for teaching cognitive skill development through newspaper or journal articles; nursing students would analyse the different viewpoints of a health-related issue, and give possible reasons for each opinion held. The use of writing, both in and out of classroom situations, has been advocated as a means of encouraging critical thinking. Lantz and Meyers (1986) describe how the skills of interpretation, analysis, elaboration, hypothetical reasoning and synthesis were developed through written accounts, followed by personification, for the teaching of pharmacodynamics and Hahnemann (1986) suggests that journal writing is a valuable tool through which reflective, analytical thinking can be fostered.

The use of problem solving has been recommended by Kurfiss (1988) as one method of helping students to develop critical thinking; she supports both Hahnemann (1986) and Lantz and Meyers (1986) by proposing the use of written formal or informal assignments or short essay questions that involve reasoning skills and the ability to organize and articulate knowledge, and the use of controversy in the form of debate, or questions presented for discussion.

These would all appear to be legitimate methods for encouraging students to develop critical thinking skills since they involve them in active learning and stimulate enquiry. However, while they are probably useful methods for developing critical thinking abilities, it is not possible to equate their implementation with the development of specific skills; a greater degree of specificity is required to delineate particular strategies which could be used by nurse teachers to promote the development of the ten key critical thinking skills assimilated by Beyer (1985a). The strategies which will be discussed are of two types: those that are deemed necessary to foster a classroom climate which is conducive to, and provides appropriate conditions for, the utilization and development of, these key critical thinking skills; and those which are linked with, and can be utilized to give students the opportunity to develop, specific critical thinking skills.

Fostering an environment for critical thinking

Baron and Kallick (1985) consider alternative ways, other than tests, to measure what is taking place in classrooms conducive to critical thinking, and ask what might be seen in a classroom where critical thinking is encouraged. They suggest that:

> first, the room is arranged so that students can see and hear each other during a discussion. Second, students are engaged with one another, and not just directing their comments to the teacher. Third, the teacher is a facilitator for students' ideas. The teacher clarifies, encourages, seeks explanations, requests illustrations and suggests alternative ideas. In other words, the teacher models the behaviour desired in students as they enter a critical thinking discussion. (p. 285)

- Planning for thinking
- Structuring the environment for student cooperation and learning
- Using appropriate questioning techniques
- Responding positively to students
- Demonstrating model thinking

Figure 4.2   Creating an environment for critical thinking: five categories of teacher activity

Costa (1985) considers that teaching for thinking requires teachers to strive to create conditions that are conducive to thinking, where they pose problems, raise questions and intervene with paradoxes, dilemmas and discrepancies that students try to resolve. In addition, they need to respond to students' ideas in such a way as to create a classroom climate that maintains trust, allows risk taking, and is experimental, creative and positive. This requires teachers to listen to students' ideas and remain non-judgemental. It is also suggested that teachers should model the behaviour desired in students (Baron and Kallick, 1985).

Glatthorn and Baron (1985) stressed the importance of the classroom climate for developing critical thinking and described what they considered to be essential elements of this process: fostering a spirit of enquiry, where the teacher feels free to admit uncertainty, welcomes intellectual challenges, and is willing to explore the unknown, as well as teach what is known, and conveys his belief in the value of thinking. There should be an emphasis on problem finding, whereby the teacher encourages the students to ask questions, as well as to answer them. Incorporating a more deliberative pace into classroom situations should discourage impulsivity and nurture the process of reflective scepticism, for which students need time to reflect on alternative possibilities, weigh the evidence and come to appropriate conclusions.

Johnson and Johnson (1979) found that cooperative work in groups promoted the use of higher reasoning strategies and greater critical thinking competencies than competitive and individualistic learning strategies. Barell (1985a) stated that teachers should spend sufficient time observing students as they listen and respond to their peers, for unless students are able to respond to the reasoning of their classmates, they will not be challenged with perspectives and solutions to problems which are different from their own. He argued that cognitive development begins to occur when, through repeated shared discussion of controversies or arguments, students begin to have cognisance of the reasoning processes of others. There is evidence that causing students to talk about their thinking processes and problem-solving strategies before, during or after their use, enhances their ability to think (Whimbey, 1985). Structured learning experiences which stimulate listening and responding help to create an environment in which communication is multidirectional, and serve to focus students not only to an answer, but to the reasoning involved in obtaining any answer, viewpoint, or question (Barell, 1985a). Brookfield (1987) considered that attentive listening enables one to take on others' perspectives and to understand others' viewpoints; it can also enable teachers to recognize when apparently incidental comments or innocuous remarks conceal powerful implicit assumptions, which can be built on as they happen, to help students realize the significance of these remarks.

Winocur (1985a) stated that higher-level cognitive objectives should be formulated when preparing for teaching so that critical thinking skills development can be coordinated, stimulated and enhanced; students need to know they will be required to engage in critical thought, and the reasons why this is important, both in the specific teaching/learning situation in which they participate and as a fundamental element of effective nursing practice. Teachers need to convey to students the goals and objectives of the session and delineate students' responsibilities for thinking (Costa, 1985). For instance, it is desirable to have multiple responses, for students to take time to respond, and for their responses to change if necessary with additional information.

Barell (1985a) identified the importance of appropriate questioning strategies in the development of critical thinking. Falkof and Moss (1984) devised a list of four types of questions which focused on the higher levels of Bloom's (1956) taxonomy, each of which required use of a different thinking skill. They found that use of these different question types by teachers, who had been trained in formulating questions, increased the incidence of higher-level answers by the students. Similarly, Malek (1986) described how the use of carefully sequenced questions encouraged students to increase and broaden their thinking and analytical skills. Careful pacing enabled students to organize their information before responding so that they offered a range of clinical alternatives for action, instead of searching for one right answer; the use of hypothetical questions enhanced students' ability to predict consequences. Lowery and Marshall (1980) considered that students are constantly anticipating how teachers will respond to their actions and the way a teacher responds is, therefore, more influential in determining students' behaviour than what he asks or tells students to do. Teacher responses that maintain, encourage and extend thinking are essential. Costa (1985) described four appropriate, open responses – using silence, or sufficient 'wait time'; accepting students' ideas and answers in non-judgemental and non-evaluative ways, so that they experience a safe psychological climate in which they can take risks and explore the consequences of their actions; clarifying students' ideas with them, so that they recognize that the teacher wants to understand fully what they are saying; and facilitating the acquisition of data by perceiving students' information needs, providing data in the form of sources of information, or making it possible for students to do so themselves, giving feedback on student performance, and surveying the whole group for input of their information.

Teachers who act as positive role models by demonstrating reflective thinking can encourage this behaviour in students. Argyris, Putnam and Smith (1985) wrote of the necessity for teachers to make their reasoning public if students are to become critically reflective by 'bringing one's views to the surface, while recognising and trying to make explicit the inferential steps that led to them' (p. 297). Exhibiting the kinds of behaviour desired in students can strongly influence their subsequent actions; being deliberate and not impulsive in responding, accepting students' differences, points of view and values, demonstrating enthusiasm about challenges and complex tasks requiring thought, and verbalizing the way in which they proceed to solve problems, are all examples of desirable behaviour discussed by Costa (1985), who also suggested that teachers should make explicit the steps they take to order statements logically within an argument and describe how conclusions are reached, and thus demonstrate the value of such deliberative activities to students when handling verbal information and written data.

Using specific strategies to promote critical thinking

The utilization of strategies which give students the opportunity to develop specific critical thinking skills depends on the teacher's conceptual understanding of critical thinking (Schwartz, 1987) and his/her ability to devise thinking skills orientated sessions through which the content of the nursing curriculum is delivered. By analysing the concept of critical thinking it is possible to distinguish four major activities in which students need to engage if they are to become competent critical thinkers, into each of which one or more of the key critical thinking skills identified by Beyer (1985a) can be categorized. These four activities and the strategies and behaviours which can be used by teachers to promote the development of specific critical thinking abilities are explored in the final section of the literature review.

First, there is a need to set cognitive tasks that require students to consider the accuracy of nursing knowledge, included in teaching sessions, and determine the adequacy and reliability of sources of data. Deliberate and clear directions concerning the cognitive tasks set are essential for students to develop an accurate perception and understanding of what they are required to do (Rosenshine and Furst, 1971). Teacher behaviours and strategies that encourage students to make sense of data and information include the use of questions and statements which ask them to work with verbal or written sources to distinguish between fact, opinion, conjecture and reasoned judgement, evaluate the soundness, factual accuracy, credibility and significance of statements, reports or findings, look for

- To consider the accuracy of nursing knowledge and determine the reliability and adequacy of sources of data
- To rationally examine and provide justification for ideas
- To verbalize and clarify their own and others' reasoning
- To use opportunities to develop reflective scepticism

Figure 4.3 Enabling students to develop key critical thinking skills: four categories of student activity

relationships between clinical data, their observations, past experiences and previous learning, consider the adequacy and relevancy of data presented, determine if additional data are required and, if so, how they could be collected, and also to validate cues or inferences they make by referring to theoretical knowledge, published research or acceptable standards (Beyer, 1985a; Ennis, 1987).

In addition, student and teacher involvement in seminars, patient-centred problem situations or case study analysis would enable students to gain practice, and develop confidence, in deciding what is of relevance and should be observed in patient situations, to derive meaning from, interpret and make clinical inferences from data, and judge the relevance and reliability of clinical findings presented (Miller and Malcolm, 1990). Competence in performing these cognitive tasks provides a foundation for the development of independent critical thought, and is a prerequisite for success in other critical thinking activities.

The second activity, the rational examination and justification of ideas, belongs at the centre of critical thinking (Ennis, 1987) but has not been encouraged in nurse education in the past, when students were tradition-ally expected to be passive recipients of knowledge imparted by teachers assuming an 'expert' role. To be accountable for their actions, registered nurses need to make explicit what they are doing and why (Clark, 1988). Therefore, strategies which ask students to support stated claims, and require them to judge the sufficiency of support for their ideas, are neces-sary. If students can justify the ideas they put forward by providing reasons to support them, it is possible for them to develop an insight into their own cognitive and affective processes (Paul, 1985). In this way, the teacher can enable students actively to monitor and regulate their use of thinking processes so that they discover automated or irrational thinking present in their subconscious thought, and identify when they need additional information or evidence to support their ideas (Costa, 1985).

It is essential to engage students in the verbalization and clarification of their own and others' reasoning if they are to become effective critical thinkers, and these processes are the focus of the third major student activity. To undertake it successfully, students need to be assisted to con-sider the ways by which they arrive at answers to problems and questions, by making explicit the stages in their reasoning; logical reasoning can be enhanced if teachers ask questions to elicit the reasoning process of students such as 'how did you arrive at your conclusion?' and by requiring students to expand on their answers (Costa, 1985; Winocur, 1985a). Ennis (1987) discussed the importance of helping students to determine the logical relationships between an author's intended meaning as they perceive it and the other meanings a statement could have. To execute the critical thinking skill of judging an argument's validity, Scriven (1976) suggested that students first have to be encouraged to clarify the meaning of words and statements used in verbal interaction and in written passages. Barell (1985a) claims that teachers who clarify and probe students' ideas and conclusions and ask them to justify their responses indicate interest and involvement through this desire to go deeper and further. Students need to be helped to determine the strengths of particular arguments and their weaknesses in terms of assumptions, biases, generalizations and ambiguities.

Finally, teachers have to ensure that their students are given opportunities to develop reflective scepticism, so that they arrive at their conclusions and convictions only after a period of questioning, analysis and reflection (Brookfield, 1987), and recognize the need for critically reflective analysis prior to making a commitment to a particular solution, idea or practice.

This activity poses a challenge both to students and teachers in nursing education since an emphasis has traditionally been placed on teaching students to do things in a preferred way that is too frequently assumed to be the one 'right' way. In addition, it has been suggested that the consequences students associate with making errors create an overwhelming fear of being wrong which makes them search for the right answer even in situations where one does not exist (Miller and Malcolm, 1990). Therefore, teachers need to discuss with students the uncertainty and ambiguity which can exist in nursing and patient care situations so that they begin to accept that there are multiple ways to achieve goals and that they will sometimes encounter problems for which the right answers are not yet known. Teachers can enhance tolerance of ambiguity by asking students for different responses, points of view and solutions, stating the acceptability of diverse responses, and recognizing the existence of multiple correct solutions (Winocur, 1985b).

By presenting students with patient-centred problems and discussing those from the students' own experience, opportunities can be created for students to suggest alternative courses of action and to predict their possible benefits, risks and consequences, prior to determining a preferred solution from the range of possibilities. Teachers who give students time to be reflective and deliberative, encourage them to search for alternatives and evaluate the consequences of their decisions, promote high quality decision making by discouraging impulsivity and decreasing the desire to achieve closure quickly (Glatthorn and Baron, 1985). Students can gain further practice in the suspension of judgement if teachers present them with different positions and responses to problematical situations in nursing contexts and ask them to analyse the arguments. In addition, where different perspectives exist, teachers should make explicit the evidence both in favour of and against each view, so that students can recognize that multiplicity and diversity of opinions and values are acceptable in the areas of nursing where knowledge is not fixed (Miller and Malcolm, 1990).

Through the exploration of alternatives, analysis of evidence and a deliberative approach to the discovery of additional possibilities, students should come to value rationality and perceive its usefulness as they problem solve, reach decisions and make judgements. Teachers should also encourage students to make a commitment to a particular position, solution or goal when the evidence and reasons for doing this are sufficient (Ennis, 1987) and be supportive towards those who, having engaged in critical reflection, wish to adopt a different viewpoint or conclusion in the light of new evidence.

Designing the tool

The measurement tool was developed from the theory base described by experts in the field of critical thinking, in which two major types of strategy were identified for the development of critical thinking skills: those considered necessary to foster a classroom climate conducive to, and providing appropriate opportunities for, the utilization and development of critical thinking skills, and those directed towards giving students the opportunity to develop specific critical thinking skills.

I ascertained that there are five categories of activity in which teachers need to engage if they are to be successful in creating an appropriate environment. These are planning for thinking, structuring the classroom environment for student interaction and cooperation, using appropriate questioning techniques, responding positively to students, and demonstrating model thinking. Within this framework, specific strategies and behaviours elicited from the literature were accommodated; these constituted 23 specific items against which the strategies used by teachers could be compared and classified.

The second type of strategy provides students with the opportunity to develop specific critical th:nking skills. Analysis of the concept of critical thinking produced four major categories of activity in which students needed to engage if they were to become competent critical thinkers: participating in specific cognitive thinking tasks, providing rational justification of ideas, verbalizing and clarifying their reasoning, and engaging in the process of reflective scepticism. Each of these categories contains at least one of the ten specific critical thinking skills identified by Beyer (1985a). Specific teaching strategies which enabled and required students to undertake these activities were extracted from the literature and matched to the appropriate category of student behaviour, yielding 27 items.

The Critical Thinking Teaching Strategies Analysis (CTTSA) tool therefore consisted of 50 specific items of teacher behaviour (see Appendix). A four-point scale was devised to measure the degree to which a teacher utilized a strategy that promoted the development of critical thinking skills within one period of teaching/learning activity, and a scoring system was allocated to the four-point scale. The scale was appropriate for all but the first two items on the analysis tool; these required a yes/no answer and were therefore rated and scored differently (Figure 4.4).

Piloting the tool

This was done to determine the adequacy of the CTTSA tool using data collected from four complete episodes of classroom teaching after obtaining consent from the teachers and students involved.

A data analysis sheet was used to record information. This listed the 50 items of teacher behaviour and, being of A3 size, had sufficient space to record relevant details.

Ten minutes prior to the scheduled start of each of these sessions, I entered the classroom setting to observe and record the arrangement of furniture at the start of the session and this was noted on the data analysis sheet. Just before the start of the session, audiotape recording was initiated, to provide an accurate aural record of verbal interaction between the teacher and the student group, and of the development of the session.

Immediately the session was completed, I returned to the classroom setting, collected and coded the audiotape and obtained copies of all written data and resources used by the teacher during the session. These included the lesson plan, handouts and acetates for overhead projection.

The use of audiotape recordings did not provide a record of silent activities, including behaviour patterns and silent actions and reactions of teacher and students (Hopkins, 1985). I recognized that visual material of the total teaching situation could have provided me with valuable additional data, but the use of a video recorder was discounted as its novelty could have disrupted normal classroom behaviour patterns, and inhibited a teacher and students unaccustomed to its presence. I rejected the idea of non-participant observation in the classroom because I thought that I would lose information if I attempted to record strategies as they occurred; the tool was too detailed to enable accurate recording of specific behaviours without the time for reflection.

Therefore, additional written information was sought to complement the audio tape recording; to obtain data about the initial structure of the

SUBJECT NUMBER:	DATE:	DURATION OF SESSION:

CRITICAL THINKING TEACHING STRATEGIES ANALYSIS TOOL

PART 1: CREATES AN ENVIRONMENT CONDUCIVE TO THE DEVELOPMENT OF CRITICAL THINKING BY:-

ITEM NO.

A. PLANNING FOR THINKING

1	Includes higher order cognitive objectives in teaching plan.	YES 3		NO 0
2	Conveys objectives for thinking to students.	YES 3		NO 0

		VERY FREQUENTLY	OFTEN	SELDOM	NEVER
3	Provides clarity and precision in verbal and written instructions.	3	2	1	0
4	Makes primary and secondary sources of information available.	3	2	1	0

ALLOCATION OF SCORES ACCORDING TO
FREQUENCY OF STRATEGY USE

ITEMS 1 AND 2 YES = 3   NO = 0

ITEMS 3–50

6 times and over	= VERY FREQUENTLY (3)
3–5 times	= OFTEN (2)
1–2 times	= SELDOM (1)
0 times	= NEVER (0)

12	Total possible score for section **A**
	Actual score obtained for section **A**

Figure 4.4 Page 1 of the Critical Thinking Teaching Strategies Analysis (CTTSA) too

classroom environment, direct observation was used. I thought that these activities would provide, at least in part, visual material for analysis.

The audiotape was transcribed and analysed, together with the lesson plan and handouts, and this information was recorded on the data analysis sheet. This information was then used to determine the teacher's rating for each item on the CTTSA tool, which enabled me to calculate section sub-scores and a total score for the teacher out of a maximum of 150.

Results from the pilot study

Total scores obtained in the four episodes investigated in the pilot study ranged from 85 to 104 (mean 95), out of a possible score of 150.

When individual scores were compared for different sections of the CTTSA tool, the highest average scores were obtained for section A (planning for thinking) and D (responding positively to students). Lowest mean scores were gained in section I (engaging students in the process of reflective scepticism) and for sections G and H (seeking rational justification of ideas and eliciting verbalization and clarification of student reasoning).

When the scores between parts 1 and 2 were compared, strategies most frequently used were directed towards creating an environment conducive to learning. Strategies which gave students the opportunity to develop specific critical thinking skills (and which require a sound knowledge of the concept of critical thinking by the teacher) were consistently used less often during the piloting of the instrument.

Issues of validity and reliability

It is important that any new measure devised is tested for reliability and validity. Face validity was assumed on the basis that the tool seemed appropriate for collecting desirable information about teaching strategies utilized by nurse teachers for the promotion of critical thinking.

Content validity is concerned with breadth of measurement, or the extent to which the items in the measurement tool are sufficiently representative of all the items that might have been selected, while construct validity relates to whether the test measures what it purports to measure (Baron, 1987).

Content validity was established by comparing the content of the measurement tool to the known literature on the topic, and validating that the tool did represent the literature accurately (Brink and Wood, 1988). The tool developed was derived from the known theory base relating to critical thinking. Therefore, I thought it reasonable to conclude that content validity had been established.

There are no other known and tested tools which measure teaching strategies utilized for the promotion of critical thinking, although Winocur (1985b) produced a Classroom Observation checklist which contains similar categories to the CTTSA tool including encouraging student interaction/cooperation, demonstrating an attitude of acceptance, encouraging students to gather information, to justify ideas and to explore others' points of view, modelling reasoning strategies, eliciting verbalization of student reasoning, probing reasoning for clarification, and encouraging students to ask questions. Individual items within some categories also correspond to a proportion of the specific items on the CTTSA tool. I was satisfied that there was a reasonable degree of consistency between them.

A few of the items on the CTTSA tool and Winocur's (1985b) checklist can also be found on a separate checklist devised by Barell (1985b). The items which appear in common on the checklists and the CTTSA tool can all be clearly traced back to the literature of these authors and others in the field of thinking and critical thinking in education. However, the checklists are not specifically developed for the purpose of measuring critical thinking strategies, but thinking in its wider sense, and so are not totally comparable with the CTTSA tool.

An acceptable method for testing the reliability of this instrument was to use inter-rater reliability as a test of equivalence, to determine if the same results could be obtained using different people to analyse the data (Abdellah and Levine, 1986). A colleague with knowledge and interest in the field of critical thinking and research expertise was asked to analyse the raw data from the piloting of the instrument, so that comparisons could be made with my analysis. No significant discrepancies were found when our individual analyses of the same data were compared for two of the teaching episodes and this provided support for the reliability of the instrument.

Final considerations

Nurse teachers are concerned with providing high quality education for nursing students with the ultimate aim of preparing professional nurses who have the ability to deliver safe, thoughtful care and can be responsive and adaptable to changing future demands. Critical thinking ability is essential if students are to function at a cognitive level which is effective for problem solving, decision making and competent clinical practice and it is too important to be left to chance.

Project 2000 (UKCC, 1986) imposed a definite requirement on nurse teachers to act on its proposals and it was this which initially prompted me to find out more about the nature of critical thinking, and how I could encourage my own students to be critical thinkers. In the course of this enquiry, I discovered that although students' ability to think critically had been investigated in the past, the process by which critical thinking was developed, and the teacher's role in this had not.

The work I undertook to fill this 'gap' in our knowledge and produce a measurement tool for the purpose was invaluable, as it required me to analyse published theoretical and research based work in both general and nursing education, and I have developed a conceptual understanding and clarity which I would otherwise not have achieved. I found that as my knowledge increased, I also began to be influenced by my reading when planning and implementing my teaching.

New ideas became incorporated into my practice; I began consciously to 'plan for thinking', revised my questioning technique and the way I responded to students. My engagement in this research activity resulted in improvements in my own teaching and this provided the motivation to continue with what seemed, at times, a daunting process for a novice researcher.

The tool has now been piloted and a formal research study can be carried out to ascertain if teachers provide opportunities for students in pre-registration nursing programmes to develop specific critical thinking skills within an appropriate environment. However, I would like to see the tool being used in a broader sense, as a tool to inform practice. For instance, it can be used by teachers in an informal way to ascertain whether they have an accurate perception of the nature of critical thinking, to provide a framework for structuring teaching/learning experiences so that they can foster critical thinking abilities, to enable teachers to communicate their expectations to students by indicating desired outcomes and levels of achievement in relation to critical thinking, and for self- and peer evaluation.

Appendix

Critical thinking teaching strategies – 50 specific items of teaching behaviour

PART 1 CREATES AN ENVIRONMENT CONDUCIVE TO THE DEVELOP-MENT OF CRITICAL THINKING BY:

A.   Planning for thinking

1.   Includes higher order objectives in teaching plan
2.   Conveys objectives for thinking to students
3.   Provides clarity and precision in verbal and written instructions
4.   Makes primary and secondary sources of information available

B.   Structuring the classroom environment for student interaction/ cooperation

5.   Provides opportunities for active participation, with students working together in pairs/groups

6.   Asks students to help others
7.   Organizes the physical environment for discussion of ideas
8.   Encourages two-way whole group interaction with teacher
9.   Allows students time to listen to and respond to their peers
10. Uses whole group for input of information

C.   Using appropriate questioning strategies

11. Provides at least 10 seconds wait time for responses
12. Gives students the opportunity to write down responses to complex questions
13. Poses questions at three highest levels of Bloom's taxonomy which require students to analyse, synthesize, evaluate, judge, predict consequences or hypothesize – 'what if', 'suppose that'
14. Requests students to pose questions

D.   Responding positively to students

15. Is non-judgemental by accepting and acknowledging all valid student responses
16. Provides encouraging, supportive comments to students with incorrect responses
17. Listens and builds on student answers
18. Provides feedback about student performance
19. Responds to student requests for information and data

E.   Demonstrating model thinking
20. Thinks aloud with students to solve problems, e.g. 'let's think this through together'
21. Solves problems in rational deliberate ways when they arise in classroom situations
22. Uses if/then language
23. Paraphrases/summarizes the logical order of statements made to reach a conclusion

PART 2   UTILIZES STRATEGIES WHICH GIVE STUDENTS THE OPPORTUNITY TO DEVELOP SPECIFIC CRITICAL THINKING SKILLS BY:

F.   Posing cognitive tasks in which student group

24. Distinguishes between fact, opinion, conjecture and reasoned judgement
25. Evaluates the soundness, credibility, factual accuracy and significance of written information, statements, reports or findings
26. Seeks relationships between clinical data, student observations, past experience and previous learning
27. Considers the adequacy/relevance of data presented

28.   Determines what additional data may be required and how they might be collected
29.   Prioritizes the data in case study/simulated problem situations
30.   States inferences obtained from interpretation of data
31.   Validates cues/inferences by reference to theoretical knowledge/published research/accepted standards

G.   Seeking rational justification of ideas

32.   Asks for evidence to support stated claims
33.   Assists student to discriminate between when adequate evidence is available and when it is not
34.   Asks students to judge the sufficiency of support for ideas by using evidence or reasoned judgement
35.   Uses 'why do you think so' questions

H.   Eliciting verbalization and clarification of student reasoning

36.   Requests students to explain the meaning of statements
37.   Asks students to elicit the reasoning behind stated claims, arguments and conclusions (of themselves and others)
38.   Invites students to make judgements and evaluations, and provide reasons for them
39.   Assists students to analyse their own answers
40.   Gives students encouragement to expand on answers
41.   Assists students to discover implicit and explicit assumptions, biases, generalizations and ambiguities in their own reasoning and that of others

I.   Engaging students in the process of reflective scepticism

42.   Requests different responses, points of view and solutions
43.   Discusses uncertainty and ambiguity in task outcome possibilities
44.   States the acceptibility of contrary responses and multiple correct answers
45.   Requests alternative courses of action to deal with patient problems
46.   Encourages students to predict the potential benefits, risks and consequences of recommendations and alternatives suggested
47.   Presents students with different positions and asks for analysis of arguments
48.   Encourages flexibility of thought by making explicit evidence in favour of and against different perspectives
49.   Requests students to determine the best alternative from a range of possiblities, giving justification for the decision
50.   Encourages and supports students to make a commitment to a position, solution, or goal, or to change an initial commitment when evidence and reasons are sufficient to do so

References

Abdellah F and Levine E (1986) *Better Patient Care Through Nursing Research*, 3rd edn. Macmillan, New York.

Argyris C, Putnam R and Smith D (1985) *Action Science: Concepts, Methods and Skills for Research and Intervention*. Jossey Bass, San Francisco.

Barell J (1985a) Removing impediments to change. In Costa A (Ed.) *Developing Minds; A Resource Book for Teaching Thinking*. Association for Supervision and Curriculum Development, Alexandria, VA, pp. 33–8.

Barell J (1985b) Appendix B: Classroom Observation Form/Appendix C: Self reflection on your teaching: a checklist. In Costa A (Ed.) *Developing Minds; A Resource Book for Teaching Thinkng*. Association for Supervision and Curriculum Development, Alexandria, VA, pp. 314–16.

Baron J and Kallick B (1985) What are we looking for and how can we find it? In Costa A (Ed.) *Developing Minds; A Resource Book for Teaching Thinking*. Virginia Association for Supervision and Curriculum Development, Alexandria, VA, pp. 281–7.

Baron J (1987) Evaluating thinking skills in the classroom. In Baron J and Sternberg R (Eds), *Teaching Thinking Skills: Theory and Practice*. W H Freeman; New York, pp. 127–48.

Bauwens E and Gerhard G (1987) The use of the Watson–Glaser Critical Thinking Appraisal to predict success in a baccalaureate nursing program. *Journal of Nursing Education* 26 (7), September, 278–81.

Beyer B (1985a) Critical thinking: what is it? *Social Education* 22 April, 270–6.

Beyer B (1985b) Practical strategies for the direct teaching of thinking skills. In Costa A (Ed.) *Developing Minds; A Resource Book for Teaching Thinking*. Association for Supervision and Curriculum Development, Alexandria, VA, pp. 145–50.

Bloom B (Ed.) (1956) *Taxonomy of Educational Objectives*. Longman, New York.

Brink P and Wood M (1988) *Basic Steps in Planning Nursing Research; From Question to Proposal*, 3rd edn. Jones & Bartlett, Boston.

Brookfield S (1987) *Developing Critical Thinkers*. Open University, Milton Keynes.

Brown L and Cook E (1971) *Selected Items for the Testing of Study Skills and Critical Thinking*, 5th edn. National Council for the Social Studies, Washington.

Clark E (1988) *Module 1: Research in Professional Development*. South Bank Polytechnic Distance Learning Centre, London.

Cohen J (1971) *Thinking*. Rand McNally, Chicago.

Costa A (1985a) Teacher behaviours that enable student thinking. In Costa A (Ed.) *Developing Minds; A Resource Book for Teaching Thinking*. Association for Supervision and Curriculum Development, Alexandria, VA, pp. 125–38.

Dressel P and Mayhew L (1954) *General Eduation Explorations in Evaluation*. American Council on Education, Washington DC.

Ennis R and Millman J (1985) *Cornell Critical Thinking Test Level Z*. Midwest Publications, Pacific Grove, CA.

Ennis R (1987) A taxonomy of critical thinking dispositions and abilities. In Baron J and Sternberg R (Eds) *Teaching Thinking Skills: Theory and Practice*. W H Freeman, New York, pp. 9–26.

Falkof L and Moss J (1984) When teachers tackle thinking skills. *Educational Leadership* 42 (3), 4–9.

Fox D (1982) *Fundamentals of Research in Nursing*, 4th edn. Appleton-Century-Crofts, Norwalk, CT.

Fraenkel J (1980) *Helping Students Think and Value; Strategies for Teaching the Social Studies*, 2nd edn. Prentice Hall, Englewood Cliffs.

Fraser D and West E (1961) *Social Studies in Secondary Schools*. Ronald Press, New York.

Frederickson K (1979) Critical thinking ability and academic achievement. *Journal of New York Student Nurses Association* 10 (1), 40–4.

Glatthorn A and Baron J (1985) The good thinker. In Costa A (Ed.) *Developing Minds; A Resource Book for Teaching Thinking*. Association for Supervision and Curriculum Development, Alexandria, VA, pp. 49–53.

Glaser E (1985) Critical thinking: education for responsible leadership in a democracy. *National Forum* 65, 24–7.

Grant G (1988) *Teaching Critical Thinking*. Praeger, New York.

Gross Y, Takazawa E and Rose C (1987) Critical thinking and nursing education. *Journal of Nursing Education* 26 (8), October, 317–23.

Hahnemann B (1986) Journal writing; a key to promoting critical thinking in nursing students. *Journal of Nursing Education* 25 (5), May, 213–15.

Hopkins D (1985) *A Teacher's Guide to Classroom Research*. Open University, Milton Keynes.

Hudgins B (1977) *Learning and Thinking*. F E Peacock, Itasca, IL.

Johnson D and Johnson R (1979) Conflict in the classroom: controversy and learning. *Review of Educational Research* 49, 51–61.

Keeley S, Browne M and Kreutzer J (1982) A comparison of freshmen and seniors on general and specific essay tests on critical thinking. *Research in Higher Education* 17, 139–54.

Kneedler P (1985) California assesses critical thinking. In Costa A (Ed.) *Developing Minds; A Resource Book for Teaching Thinking*. Association for Supervision and Curriculum Development, Alexandria, VA, pp. 276–80.

Kurfiss J (1988) *Critical Thinking: Theory, Research Practice and Possibilities ASHE-ERIC Higher Education Report No. 2*. Association for the study of Higher Education, Washington DC.

Lantz J and Meyers G (1986) Critical thinking through writing; using personification to teach pharmacodynamics. *Journal of Nursing Education* 25 (2), February, 64–6.

Lowery L and Marshall H (1980) *Learning about Instruction: Teacher Initiated Statements and Questions*. University of California, Berkeley.

Malek C (1986) A model for teaching critical thinking. *Nurse Educator* 11 (6), November/December, 20–3.

McPeck J (1981) *Critical Thinking and Education*. Martin Robertson, Oxford.

Miller M and Malcolm N (1990) Critical thinking in the nursing curriculum. *Nursing and Health Care* 11 (2), February 67–73.

Morse H and McCune G (1965) *Selected Items for the Testing of Study Skills and Critical Thinking*, 4th edn. National Council for the Social Studies, Washington.

National League for Nursing (1989) *Criteria for the Evaluation of Baccalaureate and Higher Degree Programs in Nursing*, 6th edn. NLN, New York.

Nickerson R (1987) Why teach thinking? In Baron J and Sternberg R (Eds) *Teaching Thinking Skills: Theory and Practice*. W H Freeman, New York, pp. 27–38.

Pardue S (1987) Decision making skills and critical thinking ability among associate degree, diploma, baccalaureate and master's prepared students. *Journal of Nursing Education* 26 (9), November, 354–61.

Paul R (1984) Critical thinking: fundamental to education for a free society. *Educational Leadership* 42 (1), 4–14.

Paul R (1985) Dialectical reasoning. In Costa A (Ed.) *Developing Minds; A Resource Book for Teaching Thinking*. Association for Supervision and Curriculum Development, Alexandria, VA, pp. 152–60.

Paul R (1987) Dialogical thinking: critical thought essential to the acquisition of rational knowledge and passions. In Baron J and Sternberg R (Eds) *Teaching Thinking Skills: Theory and Practice*. W H Freeman, pp. New York, 127–48.

Perkins D (1987) Thinking frames: an integrative perspective on teaching cognitive skills. In Baron J and Sternberg R (Eds) *Teaching Thinking Skills: Theory and Practice*. W H Freeman, New York, pp. 41–61.

Preseissen B (1985) Thinking skills: meanings, models, materials. In Costa A (Ed.) *Developing Minds; A Resource Book for Teaching Thinking*. Association for Supervision and Curriculum Development, Alexandria, VA, pp. 43–8.

Rhoades L and Rhoades G (1985) Using the daily newspaper to teach cognitive and affective skills. *The Clearing House* 59, 162–9.

Rosenshine B and Furst N (1971) Current and future research on teacher performance criteria. In Smith B (Ed.) *Research on Teacher Education: A Symposium*. Prentice Hall, Englewood Cliffs.

Russell D (1956) *Childrens Thinking*. Ginn and Co., Boston.

Schank M (1990) Wanted: nurses with critical thinking skills. *Journal of Continuing Education in Nursing* 21 (2), 86–9.

Schwartz R (1987) Teaching for thinking: a developmental model for the infusion of thinking skills into mainstream instruction. In Baron J and Sternberg R (Eds) *Teaching Thinking Skills: Theory and Practice*. W H Freeman, New York, pp. 106–26.

Scriven M (1976) *Reasoning*. McGraw-Hill, New York.

Shulman L (1974) The psychology of school subjects – a premature obituary? *Journal of Research on Science Teaching* 11, 319–39.

Sternberg R (1987) Questions and answers about the nature and teaching of thinking skills. In Baron J and Sternberg R (Eds) *Teaching Thinking Skills: Theory and Practice*. W H Freeman, New York, pp. 251–60.

Sullivan E (1987) Critical thinking, creativity, clinical performance and achievement in RN students. *Nurse Educator* 12 (2), March/April, 12–16.

UKCC (1986) *Project 2000: A New Preparation for Practice*. UKCC, London.

Walters J (1986) Critical thinking in liberal education: a case of overkill? *Liberal Education* 72, 233–44.

Watson G and Glaser E (1980) *Watson–Glaser Critical Thinking Appraisal: Manual*. Harcourt Brace Jovanovich, New York.

Whimbey, A (1985) Test results from teaching thinking. In Costa A (Ed.) *Developing Minds: A Resource Book for Teaching Thinking*. Association for Supervision and Curriculum Development, Alexandria, VA, pp. 269–71.

Winocur S (1985a) Developing lesson plans with cognitive objectives. In Costa A (Ed.) *Developing Minds; A Resource Book for Teaching Thinking.* Association for Supervision and Curriculum Development, Alexandria, VA, pp. 87–94.

Winocur S (1985b) Appendix F: Classroom Observation Checklist. In Costa A (Ed.) *Developing Minds; A Resource Book for Teaching Thinking.* Association for Supervision and Curriculum Development, Alexandria, VA, 322–4.

Wright E (1985) Odyssey: a curriculum for thinking. In Costa A (Ed.) *Developing Minds; A Resource Book for Teaching Thinking.* Association for Supervision and Curriculum Development, Alexandria, VA, 224–6.

5

Action on pain

Dee Burrows

This chapter clearly details the personal relevance of action research and contains a wealth of learning on the process and findings. It also:

- *discusses research when in one's own work place, offering a different perspective from Chapter 2;*
- *demonstrates clearly how reflecting on a literature review helps to form a research question;*
- *debates the modification of observation techniques to semi-participant;*
- *has a recommended list of references – a good starting point.*

The beginning of the end

Research is a confusing business encompassing lightning flashes of clarity. It is motivating with periods of despair, exhilarating but seems never to end. Even when the end does arrive there is a new beginning.

Action research envelops all these feelings, for both researcher and participants. This researcher (perhaps like others before her) is grateful that her naivete saved her from fully realizing these issues at the beginning. Without a wonderful husband, committed participants, and a consistently patient supervisor, I might never have reached the end. Or at least the end that was to be the new beginning.

Nurse teachers are in an enviable position of having a foot in the worlds of both academia and practice. Before starting my degree, I worked as a staff nurse, clinical teacher and subsequently as a link teacher on the surgical ward where the study took place. The staff were my friends and my colleagues, they motivated me, and in my way I tried to meet their needs, whether educational, professional or simply by listening.

When approached about the research, the staff quite rightly, given the existing demands of practice, wanted to know what was involved. Equally, they were keen to help and be involved. The study's aim was to introduce a pain assessment chart in an attempt to improve patients' postoperative pain management. The aim of the process was to achieve this through negotiation and partnership, strategies which are features of action research (Carr and Kemmis, 1986) as well as of my existing relationship with the ward staff.

The study took place between November 1991 and May 1992. We started by setting a standard on pain management and then undertaking educational programmes, aimed at helping us to implement the standard and pain chart in a knowledgeable and confident manner. To reduce bias and enhance the quality of data, I used methodological triangulation. The analysis suggested that the tutorials were successful in introducing the chart into clinical practice. However, I experienced problems when using observation as one of the research methods. More of that later.

The real beginning?

Life is so full of experience it is difficult to recall the real beginning. At primary school in Africa, I remember being taught basic pain physiology. The teacher used a drawing pin to indicate that a sharp prick in the buttocks resulted in a verbal cry of 'ow!'. This speedy reaction was thus pain perception. As I am sure you can visualize, the reaction of the listening seven-year-olds was one of total hilarity, but perhaps in myself there was also a spark of fascination.

My next memory was as a hospital patient. At 16, after a lovely day at my sister's first communion, I was admitted to hospital for an appendicectomy. The following days passed in a cloud of pain. My only other memory of that time was that the same doctor was always on duty – a memory that made me decide never to become a doctor! Instead, at 18 I entered nursing.

On my second ward I again faced the effect of unremitting pain. This time it was seeing a young mother, dying of metastatic breast cancer, greet her family at visiting time with smiles and hugs. Outside these hours, she was barely able to move her arms because of bone deposits. She spent what seemed like hours screaming with the pain we appeared unable to relieve. I will never forget that lady's bravery, her husband's strength, or my own feelings of helplessness.

Many other episodes impinged on my determination to do what I could to help patients in pain. As a nurse, avid reader, sometime patient and wife of a patient, I gradually formulated my ideas, and in 1988 developed the Burrows pain assessment chart (Bpac).

The chart incorporates a numerical rating scale, planning and implementation schedule, relief scale and evaluation chart. The scales, based on Hayward's (1975) painometer and Seers (1987) relief scale, have been shown to be valid and reliable in the measurement of acute pain. The planning and implementation schedule (see Figure 5.1), developed from an idea suggested by Bourbonnais (1981), correlates pain assessment scores with nursing interventions. Although Bourbonnais (1981) did not expand upon her ideas, several authors have suggested that assessment and implementation could be more closely linked (Bondestam *et al.*, 1987; Oliver, 1989).

My thoughts centred on the assumptions that all adults have past experiences of pain and may have developed pain coping strategies. Broome (1986) identified 13 cognitive and behaviourial strategies which individuals use to enhance acute pain relief, including positioning, relaxation and distraction. I felt that if nurses adopted Broome's (1986) suggestion of identifying individuals' strategies, it might be possible to continue their use in hospital. Consequently the Bpac encourages nurses to record

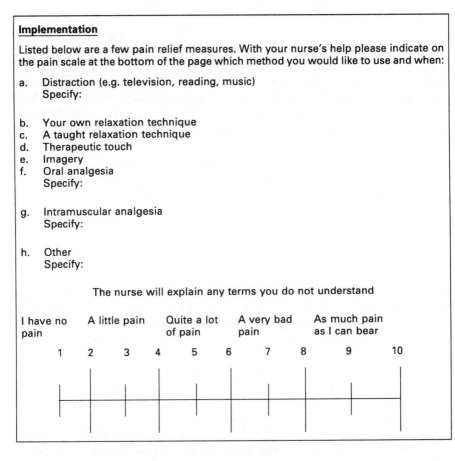

Figure 5.1   Planning and implementation schedule

patients' coping strategies, correlate interventions against projected pain ratings on the painometer, and then use this information to enhance patients' pain control.

I tested the Bpac in a small experimental study on a gynaecology ward in 1990. Statistically, small numbers allow only the most obvious effects to be detected and attempts to make generalizations may create problems (Rowntree, 1981). However, my analysis indicated that patients and nurses understood the chart, found it easy to use and effective in reducing the frequency of uncontrolled pain. Despite this it was apparent that staff were unable to utilize the Bpac fully, due to limited knowledge of interventions other than analgesia. Consequently, patients' pain coping strategies were not always incorporated into their plan of care.

Although Carr (1990a) believes that nurses are capable of implementing strategies such as relaxation and imagery without specialized input, Thomas (1991) stresses the importance of education and supervised practice to enable nurses to become skilled and confident in these techniques. My own results appeared to support the need for training. Consequently I decided that a study programme should be implemented prior to introducing the Bpac into one of the surgical wards.

Before starting the tutorials, staff wanted to develop a standard on pain management. The nurses were involved in the national RCN Standards of Care Project (Kitson, 1988) and were experienced in using the Dynamic Standard Setting System (RCN, 1990). A small group was set up comprising two staff nurses, the sister and myself.

Although standard setting can be a lengthy process, the staff's experience, together with the time I had available between meetings, enabled us to write the standard in three sessions. We considered a variety of pain assessment charts and, after discussion with the other ward nurses, decided to use the Bpac. This was one of my tensest moments – desperately wanting to use the Bpac, yet acknowledging the nurses' right to make their own decision. Without this commitment, the whole of the action research approach could have been compromised.

The standard statement was that all patients in pain would be individually assessed and their pain managed using the Bpac. The structure criteria included the production of a resource file, copies of the Bpac and the tutorial programme. Process criteria incorporated assessing patients' pain expectations and their coping strategies (if any), discussing the pain control methods available, implementing individualized pain management, and involving relatives as appropriate. Finally, the outcome criteria focused on staff stating they felt confident to use the Bpac, and patients stating they understood to expect that their pain was well controlled and the interventions appropriate.

The actual beginning

Despite my long-standing interest in pain management, I recognized that I needed to update my knowledge and clarify my more intuitive thoughts through the literature. As a teacher, I was also aware that increasing peoples' knowledge can alter their attitudes. In view of the planned tutorial programme I needed to learn more about attitudes and consider making this an explicit part of my research. Finally, I wanted to be sure that the tutorials were based on sound educational theory, so that I was not wasting the nurses' precious time, or compromising patients' quality of care.

Consequently, I make no apologies for the length of the following literature review. Rather I hope that it may act as a catalyst to encourage readers to delve further, and be critical of what follows.

Pain and pain management

Unrelieved acute pain increases psychophysiological stress, promotes immobility and delays recovery (Balfour, 1989; Carr, 1990b; Graffam, 1990). Behaviour patterns may alter and communication is interfered with. Patients may hide their pain due to fatigue, a desire to maintain dignity, or because of cultural expectations (McCaffery, 1980, 1983). Assessing and managing pain can therefore be highly problematical.

Research suggests that nurses' pain assessments are consistently at variance with those of their patients. A study by Graffam (1981) reported that 65 per cent of patients' pain ratings differed from those of nurses, while Seers (1987) found a disparity in 77 per cent of cases. Underestimating accounted for 54 per cent of these. Both authors were also concerned about the lack of effective evaluation. In Graffam's (1981) study 29 per cent of nurses believed that patients would inform them if their pain persisted, while in Seers' (1987) research this figure increased to 67 per cent. In practice, Seers (1987) found that only 37 per cent of patients asked for analgesics.

Assessing pain helps define the individual's pain experience. Yet the literature indicates that when nurses do assess pain they rely on appearance, behaviour, clinical observations and their own intuition (Graffam, 1981; Saxey, 1986; Holm *et al.*, 1989). Certainly my own observations highlighted an over-dependency on these strategies. As pain is a subjective phenomenon, it would seem more appropriate to validate inferences with the patient, through their own verbal statements (Walding, 1991). Unless nurses do this, they are unlikely to obtain an accurate picture of the person's pain (Holm *et al.*, 1989).

The use of structured pain assessment charts facilitates accurate pain assessments. Although these charts have their limitations (Jacox, 1977), research indicates that they help nurses communicate with and understand the patient's perspective (Raiman, 1986). Nevertheless not all charts are appropriate for all patients. Indeed many authors, such as Gaston Johansson and Asklund Gustafsson (1985), believe there is no one simple, practical tool available. However, the combined verbal descriptive and numerical analogue scales, devised by Hayward (1975), Bourbonnais (1981) and Seers (1987), have been shown to be reliable and easy to use. Limitations include the fact that they have only probable validity (McGuire, 1984) and may be over-simplistic in some situations.

Despite this, I believe that these scales are suited to the assessment and evaluation of postoperative pain and its relief. Not only are they quick to administer – an important point on a busy surgical ward – but they may also allow patients to self-assess. By involving patients in their own pain assessments, feelings of control can be enhanced (Walding, 1991). This, in turn, can reduce anxiety, and thereby pain perception (Hayward, 1973; Boore, 1978). Control itself can be linked to coping, as both are processes of adaptation dependent upon learning (Walker *et al.*, 1989). If individuals learn to cope and adopt strategies which facilitate control, they could be used to enhance pain management. These issues form the basic philosophy underpinning the development of the Bpac.

Before analgesics were introduced, many different methods were used to relieve pain. Most disappeared from everyday practice earlier this century, however, more recently alternative measures have increased in popularity (Astley, 1990). These vary from non-invasive methods such as therapeutic touch (Carr, 1990a), distraction (Ketchin, 1989), relaxation (Titlebaum, 1988), imagery (Vines, 1988) and music (Geden *et al.*, 1989), to invasive measures such as acupuncture (Lockstone, 1982). The former are all within the remit of nursing practice, but tend not to be used as everyday interventions. Perhaps this is because of the lack of knowledge which I uncovered in my first study.

Given that pain is a biopsychosocial phenomenon, over-reliance on analgesics as the sole relief measure may be inappropriate (Ketchin, 1989). Rather, the techniques mentioned above could be used, together with patients' own coping strategies, to enhance the effect of analgesics and improve pain control (Ketchin, 1989). To be able to do this however, nurses must be able to assess accurately, evaluate the effects of strategies systematically, and gain insight into their own personal definitions of pain and attitudes towards pain management.

Attitudes and pain management

Attitudes can be viewed from either a multi-, or unidimensional perspective. In the latter, attitudes are seen as positive, negative or neutral emotions which individuals express about an object or person (Child, 1986). Conversely, the multidimensional perspective views attitudes as a composite of cognitive, behaviourial and affective elements (Atkinson *et al.*, 1983).

Whichever perspective is taken, attitude development is influenced by many factors, including past experience, age, parental modelling and cultural expectations (Miller and Malcolm, 1990).

Katz (1960) (cited by Miller, 1979) suggests that attitudes have four major functions. The instrumental function considers the way attitudes help individuals gain rewards and avoid punishment, while the knowledge function results from people's need to create stable, organized and meaningful worlds. The value expressive category is concerned with self-concept and the adoption of group norms. Finally, the ego-defensive function relates to maintaining self-image.

The attitudes that staff develop towards pain are crucial for effective pain management. Reading Katz's (1960) (cited by Miller, 1979) work I wondered whether students' socialization into the nursing profession's norms, was directly related to the development of the many misperceptions that abound regarding pain management.

One example is nurses' fear of narcotic addiction through the over-use of analgesics. Addiction, however, is a voluntary behaviour (Long and Phipps, 1985) and studies demonstrate that the actual risk for hospitalized patients is less than 1 per cent (Marks and Sachar, 1973) (cited by Carr, 1990b). A second concern is the fear of respiratory problems. However, as Pryn (1992, unpublished) argues, patients in pain tend not to develop serious respiratory depression. Again, the likelihood is under 1 per cent.

Another common belief is that the degree of pain experienced postoperatively is directly linked to the type of surgery. Although large wounds are slower to heal and therefore uncomfortable for longer periods, there is little evidence to support this belief (McCaffery, 1983). Many nurses also regard pain experience as being age-related. While Akinsanya (1985) suggests that older people cope more easily with pain, Woodrow (1972) demonstrated that pain tolerance decreases with age. Perhaps the answer lies in Hosking and Welchew's (1985) study, where young people reported more pain and received more analgesics than the elderly.

Pain expression is also culturally bound, being learnt through primary socialization (Walding, 1991). Madjar (1984/85) compared pain behaviours in 20 Anglo-Australians and 13 Yugoslav-Australians. Although no significant differences were recorded for vocal and motor behaviours, social and verbal differences were seen. While Anglo-Australians coped by withdrawing, Yugoslavs preferred company, openly discussed their pain and yet requested less analgesics. This study was particularly interesting as I had observed a similar pattern of behaviour in patients from our local Polish community. However, such a small study should be interpreted with care, although the findings are verified by other researchers. Consequently, nurses should be aware that pain behaviours vary dramatically between cultures.

Pain tolerance on the other hand is not culturally determined. Instead it is influenced by many factors including the meaning of pain, the current emotional state (Hough, 1986), personality (Bond, 1984) and past experience (McCaffery, 1983). A study by Holm *et al.* (1989) demonstrated that nurses with intense personal pain experiences (such as myself) were more sympathetic to patients in pain than those with only mild pain experiences. They concluded that nurses must be aware of their biases and increase their knowledge regarding pain management, a piece of advice I felt I was certainly taking note of.

Education and pain management

The literature makes repeated recommendations regarding the need to improve nurses' knowledge of pain and its management (McCaffery, 1983; Raiman, 1986; Watt-Watson, 1987; Carr, 1990b; Graffam, 1990; Davis and Seers, 1991). However, Akinsanya (1985) warns that information by itself is of little value. Rather, educational programmes should address both the knowledge and attitudes required to change practice. Indeed Davis and Seers (1991) emphasize the importance of placing attitudes on the agenda of any educational programme. These comments appeared to validate my feelings that the potential for attitudinal changes, arising from the tutorial programme, should be made explicit to the staff.

In 1988 Davis undertook a study to consider the development and implementation of a pain assessment chart, concurrently with a focused educational programme. Attitudes towards postoperative pain control were tested before and after the programme to detect any changes. The results showed a significant improvement in attitudes and knowledge over the trial period. A previous study by Sofaer (1984) also demonstrated the effectiveness of ward-based teaching in improving nurses' self-awareness of their attitudes.

Ewan and White (1984) stress that several conditions are necessary for learning attitudes. These include recognition of existing attitudes, as without this individuals are working from an unknown base, provision of information which challenges these attitudes and the opportunity to test out new attitudes. All these criteria appear to have been met in the cited studies and were important considerations for my own research.

Quinn (1988) suggests that decisions about the content and process of educational programmes can be assisted by curriculum planning models. After considering those available I chose to use Beattie's (1987) Fourfold Model. This appeared particularly appropriate for devising a ward-based programme on an area as complex as acute pain management. The framework is a synthesis of several other curriculum planning approaches and is divided into four areas, addressing both the product and process of education (see Figure 5.2).

I thought that the map of key subjects, with its cognitive emphasis, would enable consideration of the biopsychosocial mechanisms of pain perception. Conversely, the portfolio of meaningful personal experiences,

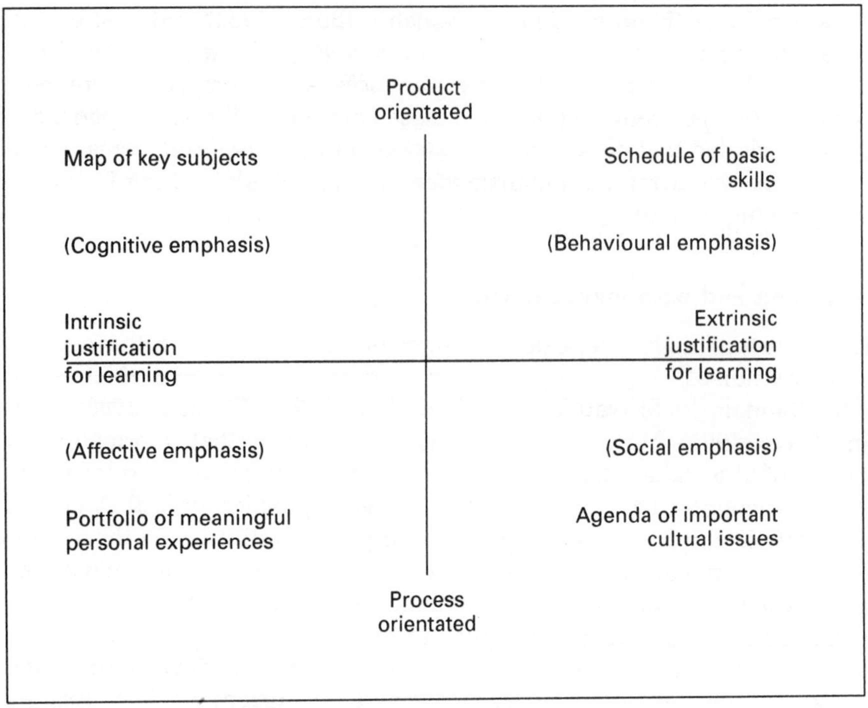

Figure 5.2   Beattie's (1987) Fourfold Model

which recognizes students' autonomy and their right to worthwhile learning, could use the nurses' own experiences to examine their attitudes towards pain and its management. The schedule of basic skills, focusing on behaviourial elements, could incorporate the skills required to use the Bpac and related interventions. Finally, the agenda of important cultural issues might act as a framework to consider the effects of current health care issues on pain management, together with explication of the attitudes that staff develop through professional socialization.

The questions

Having considered the literature and its relationship to both my previous study and the ideas I had for this study, I devised, with much help from my supervisor, the following research questions:

1   What are the attitudes of the qualified staff on the ward, towards the assessment and management of pain?
2   How effective would a series of study sessions be in facilitating attitudinal change where appropriate?

3   How effective would a series of study sessions be in facilitating the use of the Bpac in clinical practice?

Although Sofaer (1984) advocates testing patient outcomes as a method of evaluating the effects of an educational programme, my supervisor, quite rightly but sadly, persuaded me that this was too big a task to include in the time available. Consequently the results must be viewed in light of this limitation.

Answering the questions

The design I chose was action research. Like many things it is difficult to remember what prompted me first to consider this approach. I do recall comparing it with case studies, but felt these were too descriptive to meet my aims (Walker, 1983).

At the time, my main sources on action research were Cohen and Manion (1980) and a small section in Cormack (1984, see pp. 6 and 226). Since then, action research has come to the forefront of nursing research approaches, and is increasingly written about. I particularly refer the reader to Holter and Schwartz-Barcott (1993), to Christine Webb's work, one of whose references is at the end, and to Carr and Kemmis (1986). In addition anyone setting out on action research may wish to consider such concepts as empowerment, partnership and collaboration.

Cohen and Manion (1980) suggest that action research is appropriate when new direction is required within existing systems, when knowledge needs improving, or attitudes altering. On the study ward the system of pain management was rather *ad hoc*. Staff wanted to structure their approach through using a pain standard with the Bpac. They were agreeable to examining their attitudes and participating in the tutorial programme. At this level then, there was a fit between the utility of action research, my own research questions and the changes negotiated between myself and the staff.

Undertaking action research requires flexibility and continuous feedback of results (Cohen and Manion, 1980). Consequently, action research involves a cyclical process of research and action, with the aim of changing and improving practice, and increasing functional knowledge. The investigator thus acts as both researcher and change agent (Cormack, 1984).

As has previously been implied, action research requires a collaborative working relationship between researchers and participants. Although this may compromise researcher objectivity, change cannot be achieved without it (Cohen and Manion, 1980; Cormack, 1984). Of the 15 nurses involved in the study, I knew all but three of the night nurses and one day nurse, who had been appointed after I began my degree course. As mentioned earlier, I felt that I had a close relationship with the team, and perhaps particularly with the sister. I believed that this would stand me in good stead in using action research for my study.

The staff's interest in introducing the Bpac into clinical practice was a further consideration. As the literature suggests, participants must be committed to change if the researcher is to obtain feedback and innovations are to be successfully implemented (Cohen and Manion, 1980; Cormack, 1984). Conversely, the researcher must ensure that participants have sufficient information to understand the project's aims and implications. I believed that the standard setting process, together with the degree of negotiation already achieved, had gone a long way to ensuring that this was so.

I chose a variety of methods to gather data, promote change and address the research questions. I shall now briefly consider each, together with the ethical considerations involved.

Attitude scale

The attitude scale was designed to address research questions one and two. Thirty statements were compiled and presented on a five-point Likart Scale (see Figure 5.3). Half were adopted from Davis (1988), with his permission, and the remainder designed by myself. The statements were looked at by my supervisor to ensure consistency of style. Several were deliberately incorporated to assess each other, which fulfilled Duffy's (1987) criteria of 'within' method triangulation.

As with most attitude scales, many of the statements have no strictly correct or incorrect response (Davis, 1988). However, they do reflect the concerns expressed in the literature on pain and its management. I therefore believed them to have content validity (Holm *et al.*, 1989). They also reflect the composite of feelings, thoughts and behaviour about pain, consistent with a multidimensional approach towards attitudes (Atkinson *et al.*, 1983). This interpretation appeared to fit the study's aims best in explicating personal feelings about pain and its management, improving nurses' knowledge base, and enhancing the practical skills required to use the Bpac.

The questionnaire was administered prior to the standard being set, and again before and after the educational programme. This met Denzin's (1989) method of time triangulation and allowed the effects of the tutorial programme on staff's attitudes to be evaluated.

A covering letter was attached to each questionnaire assuring anonymity and asking participants to be as honest as possible. On completion the questionnaires were returned to an envelope in Sister's office for me to collect.

Educational programme

The aim of the programme was to address nurses' attitudes towards pain and to enable them to implement the Bpac in practise. To reflect the predominant attitudinal approach of the ward staff, I adopted McCaffery's (1983) humanistic definition of pain: 'pain is what the experiencing person says it is and exists when he says it does'. Unlike other definitions, which emphasize the psychophysiological aspects of pain, McCaffery's (1983) interpretation provides nurses with an operational meaning from which to practise.

Initially I asked the nurses in the standard setting group to participate in developing the content of the six, three-quarter hour sessions which were to be offered. They suggested that, as the teacher, perhaps I should use my particular knowledge and skills to do this myself. Although I was initially disappointed at this response, worrying that the collaborative nature of action research was already slipping away, I realized on reflection that the humour and tone accompanying this suggestion actually reflected a true partnership. Not only were skills being used appropriately, with me drafting the programme and the staff continuing their patient care commitments, but I also felt that the division of labour captured the true sense of collaboration.

In developing the programme I used Beattie's (1987) model in a dialectical manner, to allow for equal consideration of the four domains. I presented the draft on a poster and left it in the office for comments. I had obviously not learnt my lesson. Expecting to make changes, I was taken by surprise when the nurses said it looked very appropriate, and I obviously did know what they needed! Further speedy reflection made me realize that my personal knowledge of the nurses, the client group, and the ward itself, had left me in a good position to accurately identify their needs. The programme content is shown in Figure 5.4 and detailed below:

1) The Standard and Related Research: Initially the nurses outside the standard setting group needed to know about the standard and the research we had considered in developing it. The session was therefore rather teacher-centred, although participants were encouraged to be critical and objective.

2) The Meaning of Pain: We discussed the results of the first two attitude questionnaires, focusing upon those attitudes contradicted in the literature, together with the influence of society and nursing's culture on individuals' attitude development. Participants left the session with a handout on the related research for further consideration.

3) The Bpac: In this session I provided an overview of the development of the Bpac, including the assumptions underpinning it and the research previously carried out. A demonstration of its use was given, followed by supervised practice on one another. Each nurse was given a heat-sealed copy of the pain and relief scales, together with a copy of the chart.

	Strongly Agree	Agree	Unsure	Disagree	Strongly Disagree
1. Nurses can determine accurately the amount of pain a person will suffer from knowledge of the surgery.					
2. Talking to patients preoperatively about pain helps reduce pain post-operatively.					
3. Analgesics are always the best way of reducing pain.					
4. Using pain assessment charts provides a more accurate picture of the patient's pain.					
5. All real pain has an identifiable physical cause.					
6. Education on pain management helps nurses recognize when patients are in pain.					
7. It is best that patients should not know what is happening to them as this may cause anxiety.					
8. Patients who have had surgery (of any type) in the past, know what to expect with regard to postoperative pain.					
9. Patients should expect to suffer some pain.					
10. A person's age affects their tolerance to pain.					
11. Anxiety increases the perception of pain.					
12. Patients complaining of pain 2-3 hours after an injection should be encouraged to wait a little longer for their next injection.					
13. Nurses most often underestimate the severity and existence of a person's pain.					
14. Patients who refuse analgesics when they are in pain are not acting in their own best interests.					

Figure 5.3 Attitude scale to pain management. Odd numbered questions and question 30 taken from Davis (1988)

	Strongly Agree	Agree	Unsure	Disagree	Strongly Disagree
15. Some ethnic groups can tolerate more pain than others.					
16. It is possible to control pain post-operatively					
17. Talking and listening to patients can reduce their pain.					
18. Patients should receive postoperative analgesics on a PRN basis only.					
19. Nurses always make accurate inferences about the severity and existence of a person's pain					
20. Relaxation and distraction techniques are effective measures in relieving pain					
21. The person who uses his/her pain to obtain benefits or preferential treatment does not hurt as much as he/she says he/she does and may not hurt at all.					
22. Patients should receive postoperative analgesics on both a regular and PRN basis.					
23. What the person says about his/her pain is always true.					
24. Patients who refuse analgesics show a great sense of character.					
25. Nurses are better qualified and more experienced to determine the existence and nature of a person's pain than the person him/herself.					
26. Patients should receive analgesics on a regular basis only.					
27. All persons can and should be encouraged to have a high tolerance to pain.					
28. Nurses learn enough about pain during their training to manage patient's post-operative pain effectively.					
29. Care should be taken when giving controlled drugs postoperatively as patients easily become addicted.					
30. A person's pain can always be detected by their behaviour and physiological signs.					

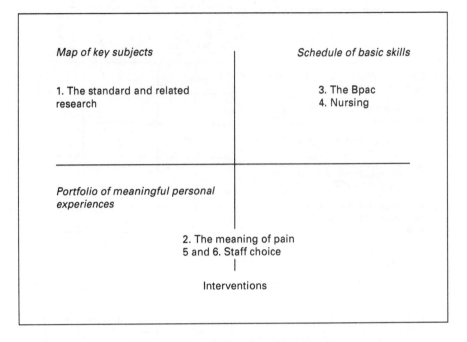

Figure 5.4 The Fourfold Model applied to the educational programme

4)   Nursing Interventions: This was a practical session where we all shared our knowledge on a variety of interventions. Demonstrations were incorporated as appropriate and discussions related to the utility of the intervention for the ward's particular client group and environmental setting. My own role was that of coordinator, together with demonstration and supervision of guided imagery and therapeutic touch.

5) & 6)   Staff Choice: The content of these tutorials was negotiated at the time. The first focused on further nursing interventions, and the second on individual problem solving.

I managed to present each tutorial twice a week to maximize the opportunity for staff to attend. I displayed a poster detailing dates, times and session titles. I also specifically informed the night staff and invited them to attend if they were free. In addition I organized two, one-and-a-half hour sessions at night, focusing upon the content of tutorials one and three. These were exceptionally well attended as the night sister organized relief for the study ward's staff, and also freed up a nurse from almost every other ward in the hospital. It certainly made up for my loss of sleep, as well as reflecting the night staff's commitment to pain management. Perhaps more sadly, I also felt that it demonstrated the hunger for further education, tailored to the working lives of those devoted to providing quality patient care at night.

Finally the nurses kindly agreed to allow me to tape the tutorials. Not only did this provide data on participants spoken attitudes, which could then be compared to those recorded on the attitude scales (Denzin, 1989), but it also enabled me to produce a learning package for new and existing staff.

Interviews

The interviews provided data on participants' feelings about the standard and Bpac, the effects of the tutorial programme on their knowledge and attitudes, and the action research approach.

I chose to use semi-structured interviews as they appeared to allow a balance between control and openness and seemed useful in determining attitudes and perceptions (Cohen and Manion, 1980). To maintain the balance, I adopted Nisbet and Watt's (1980) suggestion of compiling a schedule to act as a guide.

The interviews themselves were carried out with six of the day staff, who consented to be interviewed and were on duty at the times I was able to visit. Knowing them as well as I did, I was concerned about the risk of leading participants through verbal and non-verbal cues (Treece and Treece, 1986). Consequently I tried to maintain a 'neutral' expression and tone, while being friendly and attempting to relax them. I obtained permission to use a tape recorder, and again followed Nisbet and Watt's (1980) suggestion of transcribing key statements, with quotations only when appropriate.

Observation

The planned observation focused on the ability of four of the day staff to use the Bpac in practice. However despite being aware of the potential difficulties of using semi-participant observation, I was only able to gather objective data from two of the four participants. Given the difficulties I experienced, I have chosen to critique this area of my study in greater depth later in this chapter.

Ethical considerations

When planning my initial research on the Bpac, I submitted a full proposal to the District Ethics Committee stating my intention of introducing the chart to other wards in the surgical unit, at a later date. As a result of this, and the fact that I had no plans to obtain data directly from patients, the Chairman of the Committee granted permission for this project, following an informal discussion of its parameters.

I also approached the Director of Operational Services and appropriate senior nurse to gain their consent, as well as seeking formal agreement from each of the participants. Finally, I contacted the researcher for the

RCN Standards of Care Project, as I was concerned that my study should not interfere with the national project. In fact, she believed that the study would help the team to take responsibility for standard setting. Consequently she kindly gave her permission.

I assured staff of confidentiality through anonymity of the attitude scales, by destroying all tapes immediately after transcribing, and ensuring that participants' names did not appear on the transcripts. The interviews took place in a private area, with only myself and the individual nurse present.

The answers

To reflect the humanistic nature of the research I have presented my findings in an integrated format with the discussion and limitations. The main areas identified were: staff attitudes; the standard and Bpac; the educational programme; and staff and researcher perceptions of the action research process.

Of the 15 attitude scales distributed, 11 were returned on the first and third occasions, and nine on the second. The response rate was thus 73 per cent and 60 per cent respectively. Given my relationship with the staff you may wonder why the return was not 100 per cent. In fact I was tremendously pleased with the response. Because only two weeks elapsed between each distribution and the required return date, there were always staff on holiday, study or sick leave. Furthermore, I know of at least one nurse who, although completing the scales, declined to submit them for analysis. This participant's choice was respected and no effort was made to identify her reasons. Possibly it was because she is a very private person, who at the time was also experiencing a lack of confidence in her overall knowledge level.

Nine day nurses were eligible for the interviews, however, two were unavailable on the day and a third declined to be involved. The remaining six staff agreed to participate. Four staff volunteered to participate in the observations.

Staff attitudes

The data obtained from the attitude scales, tutorial tapes and interview transcripts showed that the nurses' attitudes were generally consistent with those recognized as appropriate in the literature. To assist my analysis six theme clusters were identified, each of which is addressed in turn.

Pain perception

This was one of the few areas in which participants' attitudes differed widely from the literature. For example, when asked whether 'all real pain has an identifiable cause', three initial respondents believed that it does, while a further nurse was unsure. Nine nurses thought that age affected pain perception, while six believed that 'some ethnic groups are able to tolerate more pain than others'. A further two were unsure of this statement.

Despite the educational programme there was little alteration in these attitudes over time. I was particularly disappointed in the lack of change regarding the cultural statement, as I had spent a lot of time on this issue. Given the local population of Asians and Polish nationals, as well as Anglo-Saxons, a variety of pain behaviours are seen on the ward. Although staff were aware of the behaviours adopted by Asians, they were less clear of the Polish patients' strategies.

I presented Madjar's (1984/85) research on cultural pain behaviours during the tutorials, and we discussed the possible links between the coping strategies used by Yugoslav-Australians, and those exhibited by the ward's Polish patients. Although staff found the study interesting, and appeared to see the relevance for their clinical practice, only four respondents in the final questionnaire agreed that pain perception is not culturally determined.

Possibly some nurses found it difficult to differentiate between pain tolerance and pain behaviour. Although this statement was adopted from Davis' (1988) scale, it may need rewording to remove any latent ambiguity. A further explanation is that only four of the nine day staff were able to attend the relevant tutorial, due to sickness and annual leave.

Pain tolerance

My only area of concern regarding pain tolerance, related to the statement 'patients should expect to suffer some pain'. Initially eight nurses agreed with this statement with a further two being unsure. However, these figures fell to five and one respectively following the second attitude recording. Again I paid considerable attention to this attitude during the tutorials. Some improvements were seen, with those disagreeing with the statement increasing from one at the first recording, to four on the last. However, five nurses continued to maintain their beliefs.

Statements from the tutorial transcripts indicated that staff believe it is healthy to experience pain, that pain is needed for endomorphin release and that some patients need to feel pain to know they are alive. Not only are these attitudes contradicted by the literature, which indicates that pain adversely affects recovery (Carr, 1990b), but they are also worrying in the light of Seers' (1987) research, which demonstrated that the more pain patients experience, the lower they themselves rate their recovery. In addition they show little regard for the ICN's (1973) directive that nurses have a responsibility to alleviate suffering.

One nurse however commented that she now uses McCaffery's (1983) operational definition, although at times she finds this difficult. She also stated, 'I didn't feel before all this that you could realistically aim for a patient to be completely pain free. I think it's a hard goal but I now feel it is achievable'.

While I found this comment rewarding and refreshing, I believe that the nurses need more or perhaps better education on this issue. Unfortunately my concerns with wiping the tapes after transcribing meant that I was unable to return to the tape to evaluate my own teaching ability on this point. I am left with a feeling of not knowing whether it was 'my fault, or not'.

Anxiety and pain

All participants agreed that anxiety increases pain perception and that preoperative information-giving helps to reduce postoperative pain. Several factors existed that may have influenced this positive approach, including a study carried out on the ward one year prior to my own, which considered the provision of preoperative information (Grace, 1990, unpublished). More recently staff set a standard on information-giving.

Pain assessment

To my relief all the nurses acknowledged that they are less well qualified to determine the nature of pain than the patient themselves. The majority also believed that staff do not always make accurate inferences about pain, while seven respondents to each questionnaire agreed that nurses underestimate pain. However, two disagreed with this statement and a further two were unsure. These figures did not alter following the tutorials.

In her study Seers (1987) found that 33 per cent of nurses assessed pain accurately, while a further 13 per cent tended to overestimate pain. It is feasible that the nurses disagreeing with the last statement fell into one of these two categories. Of course it is equally conceivable that they did not. However, it was impossible to discover this due to the anonymity of the attitude questionnaire. Indeed I found this to be a repeated frustration and constraint, although I still believe that the answers were more likely to be honest because of the anonymity. Even so, the temptation to code the later questionnaires, to identify individuals, was difficult to resist.

Worryingly, a significant number of respondents in the first and third questionnaires (six and five respectively) believed that pain can always be detected by behavioural and physiological signs. Again for reasons that could not be determined, only one nurse recorded this response to the second questionnaire. Because pain is exhausting and the body is able to adapt physiologically, the existence of pain cannot always be determined on the above basis (McCaffery, 1980; Roy, 1984). Equally, as previously mentioned, cultural expectations will influence patients' pain behaviour (Madjar, 1985).

The views expressed here appeared to contradict the participants' belief that 'what the person says about his/her pain is always true'. If patients' verbal statements are to be accepted, nurses cannot qualify this with expectations of behavioural and physiological signs. The apparent inconsistency of these attitudes may reflect dissonance between staff's conative intentions and their cognitive beliefs.

The statement 'using pain assessment charts provides a more accurate picture of the patient's pain' was agreed with by ten of the 11 initial respondents and remained consistent over time. During the tutorials one participant stated that 'a pain chart is probably more important than the TPR and B/P chart', while another commented that 'patients are very reluctant to tell us what their pain is' without the use of a chart. This finding, together with the previously expressed belief that nurses do not make accurate inferences about pain, suggested that staff were highly motivated to use pain assessment charts.

Pain relief interventions

To use the Bpac, nurses must be able to implement a variety of interventions. Staff thus needed sufficient knowledge and commitment to do so. The results of the final attitude questionnaire suggested that this was the case. Only one respondent expressed uncertainty on the effectiveness of relaxation and distraction, while all staff acknowledged the benefits of talking and listening. Indeed one commented, 'we actually need to recognize it's an intervention'. A further participant believed that pain management is 'really (about) identifying how people are coping with their pain'.

However, when asked whether 'analgesics are always the best way of reducing pain', one respondent in the first and second recordings thought they were, while two expressed this opinion following the tutorials. When properly administered, analgesics may be effective for a large number of patients, however, alternative interventions are a useful adjunct to medication and to enhance patients' perceptions of control (Ketchin, 1989).

The interview data indicated a major shift towards the deliberate use of non-analgesic measures. Those mentioned by two or more staff included guided imagery, therapeutic touch, relaxation and talking. Positioning, distraction, warm baths and ice were also listed, while music therapy was viewed as an intervention for future development. It appears from these findings that nurses need to learn actively about these strategies if they are to implement them confidently. Consequently, I firmly disagree with Carr's (1990a) opinion that nurses are capable of utilizing such techniques without training.

Analgesic administration

A study carried out at the hospital by Pryn (1992, unpublished), the results of which were released two weeks into the tutorial programme, may well have influenced the positive findings in this category. A major part of the study focused upon the misconceptions of narcotic addiction, and the importance of administering analgesics on both a regular and PRN basis. The report was read by us all and discussed in the tutorials. In the interviews one nurse stated that since the tutorials she now offers medication, rather than waiting for patients to ask for it. Another commented that she has become particularly aware of the amount of Oromorph given to terminally ill patients for break-through pain, resulting in several MST regimens being reviewed.

The only contradictory finding in this cluster related to the statement, 'patients who refuse analgesics when they are in pain are not acting in their own best interests'. In the first questionnaire, two nurses were unsure of their opinion and two disagreed with this statement. In the second, the figures were one and two respectively, while the third questionnaire resulted in four nurses disagreeing. I found these results puzzling, as the nurses appeared to be aware that uncontrolled pain causes immobility, increasing the risks of deep vein thrombosis, urinary retention, pneumonia and pressure sores (Carr, 1990b; Graffam, 1990). A possible explanation is that two of the nurses clarified the meaning of this statement with me. Perhaps those who disagreed found the wording ambiguous.

The educational programme

Attendance at the tutorials varied according to patient care commitments and participants' off-duty. Although all staff were present at the sessions on the Bpac, individual attendance at the remaining daytime tutorials, varied from 0 (1 subject) to 83 per cent (2 subjects).

At times this was extremely frustrating and I reflected this in my field notes, which occasionally acted as a private medium for me to pour out my feelings without upsetting anybody else! The conflict of researcher versus nurse, appreciating the demands of practice, was particularly difficult. My saving grace was once again my relationship with the nurses and particularly the ward sister who seemed to pick me up on numerous occasions. Equally my other 'support personnel' worked overtime at this stage, never knowing whether I would be exhilarated because everything was going well, or down-hearted because I was struggling. Such is the fascination of research.

The nurses found the tutorials helped them to understand the standard and Bpac and increase their functional knowledge of pain management. Although most felt they had a reasonable knowledge before the tutorials started, five of the six interviewees commented that this had improved during the programme. Two also suggested that pain is an area they need to continue 'reading up on', while four stated that they discussed their knowledge and attitudes outside the tutorials and had become more aware of the issues involved in pain management. One commented, 'everybody gets complacent and you start to look at things again that maybe you were beginning to close your eyes to'.

As the programme progressed, attitudes regarding the adequacy of pre-registration education on pain altered. Initially, two respondents believed this to be sufficient and one was unsure. However, following the tutorials only one nurse maintained this opinion. These findings suggest that staff became increasingly aware of the complexity of the topic and amount of knowledge required to nurse patients in pain.

Participants also commented that following the tutorials they had become aware of incorporating pain management deliberatively into care plans, and of discussing pain relief with other health professionals immediately the need arose.

The standard and Bpac

With one exception, the more tutorials nurses attended the more confident they were in using the Bpac. The exception was a nurse who wished to see the chart used with a patient, prior to implementing it herself. She stated, 'it actually terrifies me using it with the patient – the explanation and getting it over clearly. Once it becomes everyday practice though, it'll be alright'. This nurse had been present at four of the six tutorials, missing one on nursing interventions, and the final tutorial where problems were discussed on an individual basis. Of all the participants I was particularly surprised by this nurse's feelings. Not only was she an experienced member of the staff, but was also generally quite confident. However, she is known as a perfectionist and it may have been this which caused her feelings.

Five of the six interviewees planned to continue using the standard. The auxiliary nurse, however, felt unable to do so because of her lack of knowledge and qualifications. This also affected her ability to use the Bpac. Of the remaining nurses, four had implemented the Bpac with selected patients. All believed that the chart enhanced the assessment and management of pain, by improving nurse–patient communication, facilitating the use of a variety of strategies, increasing patient involvement, and enabling nurses to evaluate the effectiveness of their interventions.

The area in which participants had the most difficulty was in assessing patients' own coping strategies when first introducing them to the chart. As well as a natural reticence to change, staff feared that some patients 'find it quite hard to become involved' and that this causes them to question the nurse's knowledge. I had opted for simulations within the office to enhance safety during learning and enable immediate problem solving. With hindsight, while this was useful, additional demonstrations involving patients should have been offered to each nurse individually. Despite this, the overall result of the tutorial programme was the successful implementation of the Bpac.

Staff and researcher perceptions of the action research process

Action research helps to close the gaps between practice, education and research (Cohen and Manion, 1980). In this study, it also appeared to be effective in promoting innovative change.

The attitudinal changes seen following the tutorials were less dramatic than those found by Sofaer (1984). Her study involved 80 nurses on five wards, with data collection spread over one and a half years. Consequently she was able to offer each tutorial on more than two occasions, ensuring that all nurses completed the programme. Unfortunately, I was unable to do this because of other commitments.

A second issue was that, overall, nurses participating in my study already held positive attitudes towards pain and its management. Consequently, I did not expect dramatic changes. However, staff did gain insight into their attitudes and recognized the changes that occurred. I was particularly interested in one nurse who, unable to attend the tutorials, photocopied the scales to monitor her attitude changes. She believed that these occurred as a result of being forced to acknowledge her attitudes when completing the scales. This process appears consistent with Ewan and White's (1984) theory regarding the conditions necessary for attitude learning.

Many of the ward's nurses have particular expertise in certain interventions. The educational programme allowed this expertise to be made explicit, and shared throughout the team. To me this seemed to reflect the partnership and collaboration that is so central to action research. Equally, the sucessful implementation of the standard, Bpac, and the interventions themselves, highlighted the utility of this approach in promoting changes in practice. However, if these changes were to be sustained, staff needed to use the chart regularly and have a forum available to discuss problems. Consequently, we agreed to hold six-monthly formal follow-up sessions. Although these were maintained for 18 months, changes in my own role prevented me from continuing them. However, a copy of the learning package and resource file remain available on the ward.

The critical scrutiny to which participants have to subject themselves makes action research a stressful process (Cormack, 1984). Equally, the change process itself increases both anxiety and workloads. To reduce these negative effects, participants must be clear about the research goals and committed to their achievement (Cohen and Manion, 1980). During the third week of the educational programme I began to feel that one of the nurses lacked understanding of the research. Her motivation was affected, and she appeared to influence others towards a lack of commitment to the tutorials.

The Sister and I had an open and productive talk and decided on several strategies. These included Sister discussing the study's progress with the staff, while I wrote to them thanking them for their support and announcing that we were over halfway there. I also acknowledged that this nurse was the only qualified member of the team who knew me solely as a visiting researcher. Consequently, we agreed that I would work on the ward during a shift when she was in charge. As the morning progressed, it became evident that I was becoming clinically credible in her eyes. The rather dramatic outcome was total commitment from this nurse, who, indeed, became one of the driving forces for the remainder of the study.

This experience clearly illustrates the importance of clinical credibility in forming collaborative working relationships when using action research. It is a theme that has been addressed by Webb (1990) and one that I personally will never forget. Indeed I still find my field notes, written in the form of a diary at this time, totally fascinating. As teachers, it is easy to forget that others may not see our commitment to clinical practice, unless we actually 'do it'.

Using and abusing semi-participant observation

As mentioned earlier, because of the problems I experienced with using observation, I have chosen to look at this area in more depth. Some of these problems arose as a result of my lack of preparation, and I hope that you will find this discussion helpful in preventing you from making the same mistakes!

Observational approaches

Observation is a systematic approach to collecting data through observing and recording behaviour (Polit and Hungler, 1987). Unlike other methodologies, observational studies are centred within participants' natural settings (Cormack, 1984; Murphy and Albers, 1992). Observers can be known or unknown. The latter creates considerable ethical problems and is often discredited by researchers (Treece and Treece, 1986). Conversely, known observers can bias findings through the 'Hawthorne effect', whereby subjects may alter their performance as a result of being the centre of attention (Wainwright, 1990).

Three main types of observation exist: participant, semi-participant and non-participant (Bailey, 1987; Reid, 1991). Participant observers become part of the group they are studying. They are thus able to gain an understanding of the situation from the inside. However, it may be difficult to combine systematic observations with role performance. Issues and events can leak away and subjectivity is an ever existing danger (Bailey, 1987; Wainwright, 1990). Furthermore, observers using this approach may end up 'going native', by refuting their researcher role and becoming fully socialized group members (Cohen and Manion, 1980). This may arise as a result of fascination with the group, or perhaps because the researcher has previously been a member of the group. An example of the latter is the nurse teacher carrying out research in an area where she has clinical expertise.

Non-participant researchers act as spectators. They are thus able to focus on collecting data without the distractions of a secondary role. However, artificial situations can arise and aspects of interactive behaviour may be missed (Wainwright, 1990). Conversely, semi-participant observers visit the group frequently and become involved, but not immersed, in the culture (Reid, 1991). Advantages of this approach include being able to maintain a degree of objectivity, while observing interactive behaviour closely. Depending upon the balance of observation versus participation, the dangers of either of the previous approaches may exist.

Murphy and Albers (1992) describe three further types of observation: cohort, case-control and cross-sectional. The first two are quantitative in approach and readers are referred to the original paper for further explanation. Cross-sectional studies focus upon concurrent measurement of interventions and outcomes in a preferably random population sample. Cause and effect cannot be determined, although trends may be evident. Cross-sectional studies tend to lack depth but may be useful for evaluating educational programmes.

Rationale for the choice of semi-participant observation

Including observation as a methodology fulfilled Duffy's (1987) suggestion of 'between' method triangulation, whereby I could cross-check data obtained from both the interviews and observations, for evidence relating to the third research question: 'How effective would a series of study sessions be in facilitating the use of the Bpac in clinical practice?'. While interviews obtained data on what participants said about their ability and confidence, observation enabled me to gain insight into what they actually did (Strong, 1979, cited by Reid, 1991).

In choosing which type of observation to use, I felt that a non-participant style would be inappropriate for several reasons. First, given the research question it was important to gain insight into participants' interactive behaviour as a measure of their skill and confidence in using the Bpac. Equally, my familiarity with the staff, and the collaborative nature of action research, would have made adopting a spectator's role both uncomfortable and unnatural. Surprisingly perhaps, it was precisely this familiarity that dissuaded me from using participant observation. The risk of going native and losing objectivity appeared all too likely. Furthermore, I needed to ensure that it was the nurses' skills, rather than my own, that were being evaluated.

I thus adopted a cross-sectional, semi-participant approach. I viewed the tutorials as the intervention and participants' ability to use the Bpac with confidence, as the tested outcome. As a frequent visitor to the ward over a period of several years, I saw myself as being involved in both the professional and social culture, without being totally immersed on a daily basis. My main concern was that I could become more involved than initially intended. However, at the time, I believed, somewhat naively, that being aware of this problem would prevent it happening!

Implementing semi-participant observation

A representative sample of the day staff were involved in the observations, including the F grade nurse, an experienced E grade and two D grade nurses. Each was on duty at the times I was able to visit and I asked them in advance whether they would participate.

Although all staff had originally consented to the study I felt it was important to gain separate informed consent for each of the data collection methods. Being observed can be highly stressful and this is particularly so when learning and ability are being evaluated. The staff were given explanations regarding my role as a semi-participant observer, and the behaviours being observed. Opportunities for feedback were offered.

Both Reid (1991) and Cannon (1989) discuss fears of intrusion during observational studies. However, in talking to staff the impression I gained was that while participants acknowledged the research element, they also viewed the observations as an opportunity to continue their learning in a controlled and supportive environment. Furthermore, they appeared keen to 'show off' their skills. I found these comments highly motivating and again they seemed to reflect the action research philosophy.

As a research methodology, observation was a new experience for me. However, Wainwright (1990) suggests that nurses are generally skilled observers and he advocates increasing the use of this approach in nursing research. This, together with discussing my plans with my supervisor, and reading several papers on observation, gave me confidence.

Bailey (1987) suggests that observation can be either structured or unstructured, although the distinction between the two may at times be unclear. Cormack (1984) and Treece and Treece (1986) both advocate the use of schedules to record observations, and coding systems to direct analysis. However, Reid (1991) believes that such structure can prove constricting. Both she and Bailey (1987) discuss the use of unstructured field notes as a method for descriptive recording and reflection. It was this perspective that I adopted, as it appeared to be more suited to both semi-participant observation and to collecting data on ability and observed confidence. I planned to write the notes up immediately following each observed event.

I worked on the ward, in uniform, for two days. During this time participants self-selected the observation events, requesting my presence as appropriate. As my area of interest was confined to the nurses' use of the Bpac, constant observations would have been time-consuming, stressful and unnecessary. The behaviours I observed and recorded in my field notes included the clarity of explanation, readiness to answer patients' questions, eye contact between the nurse and patient, the patients' facial expressions and nurses' reaction to these, the depth of recordings made on the Bpac and the appropriate use of clients' coping strategies. Participants were observed at initial assessment and explanation of the chart with preoperative patients, and also in pain management events with postoperative patients.

Research versus change

I observed postoperative events with all four nurses. Each was using the painometer, relief scale and a variety of nursing interventions accurately and confidently. Recordings were in sufficient depth to reflect the event, and provide information for other members of staff involved in the patient's pain management.

Two nurses were observed explaining the chart, assessing coping strategies and correlating these against projected pain ratings. Both were clear and comprehensive in their explanations, completing the full assessment in approximately 10 minutes. Participants stated they felt comfortable and confident with their technique, and believed that the time would be reduced as they became more skilled.

The remaining nurses clearly lacked confidence in explaining the planning and implementation schedule. Through skilled use of non-verbal communication, they 'requested' my help early in the event, a strategy that was positively evaluated in the feedback. I thus adopted a participant approach, giving the support required. Following this, both nurses said they felt sufficiently confident to use the schedule. Unfortunately I was not able to observe these nurses again.

Reflecting on my field notes raised a number of issues. Both these nurse were D grade staff nurses and it may be they lacked confidence in their clinical practice. Furthermore, I had known them as students, which could have stopped them relaxing. As Reid (1991) states, subjects may feel they are being observed for what is right or wrong about their behaviour. Their perceptions of my status, together with my obvious familiarity with the Bpac, may also have led them to abdicate responsibility. Finally, both had a relatively low attendance at the tutorials (50 per cent each), due to sickness, study and annual leave.

Despite being aware of the risk of becoming involved, this is precisely what I did. Through acknowledging the nurses' expressed needs, I, as the researcher, or in this instance the change agent, used role modelling to facilitate further learning. Although this compromised objectivity and the systematic collection of data, I believe that it actually enhanced the change process inherent in action research. Consequently I felt that my actions benefited the study as a whole.

However, I also felt that the techniques I used to plan, conduct and analyse the observations were not as systematic as they might have been. This was partly due to my lack of experience and the increased level of participation, but perhaps of greater concern I came to realize that I was insufficiently prepared mentally.

Given that all research is constrained by time, there is a danger that new researchers will be limited in the amount they can learn in relation to their approach and methodology. This is particularly so if a variety of strategies are used to achieve methodological triangulation. With hindsight, I recognize that I paid least attention to reading about observation, as it appeared the smallest and quickest element of the study. I also feel that because it was the last method I employed, my attitudinal approach was less committed. It was also all too easy to 'go native', and adopt a clinical teaching role.

Subsequent reading and learning has highlighted both the positive and negative points in using this strategy, many of which are contained in this critique. I also appreciate how lucky I was not to experience considerably more difficulties. In the future, I will seek advice on adopting a more deliberative, controlled and systematic approach.

A new beginning

Because action research is situation specific, direct generalizations cannot be made to the larger population. However, Sandelowski (1986) argues that the researcher can indicate 'applicability'. As such, I believe that the standard, educational programme and Bpac could be adopted by other wards in the surgical unit, as long as the tutorials are developed to meet individual needs.

So where do I go from here? The answer of course is into the new beginning. The assumptions underlying the Bpac need investigating. Perhaps the starting point needs to be in identifying whether or not people do actually use coping strategies to manage their own acute pain. Even if they do, would they use them in hospital, and could we support them? Some of the answers have been indicated by my two studies so far. Nurses implementing the Bpac have identified strategies that people use, and they have supported this use within an acute surgical setting. However, the benefits, if any, of doing so, have clearly not been systematically evaluated with patients. This then is the new beginning.

Meanwhile, if patients' pain is to be controlled, nurses must assume the responsibility for relieving pain. To achieve this, education needs to give a higher priority to the assessment and management of pain, and encourage nurses to adopt quality assurance measures in their clinical practise. Educationalists and practitioners must therefore work together to provide the standard of pain control to which every patient has a right.

Acknowledgements

I would like to thank all the nurses who so generously gave of their time, Pam Robinson and Sue Grace for their invaluable advice and help, and my college facilitator Alan Myles for his unfailing patience. Special thanks are offered to Peter Davis who kindly agreed to the use of his attitude scale, and to Sally Thomson for her motivating influence in the writing of this chapter. Lastly I wish to thank my husband, Mick, for his unfailing support and assistance with the initial development of the Burrows pain assessment chart, the research itself, and the production of this chapter.

References

Akinsanya C Y (1985) The use of knowledge in the management of pain: the nurse's role. *Nurse Education Today* 5(1), 41–6.

Astley A (1990) A history of pain. *Nursing: The Journal of Clinical Practice, Education and Management* 4, 23 September, 33–5.

Atkinson R L, Atkinson R C and Hilgard E R (1983) *Introduction to Psychology.* Harcourt Brace Jovanovich, New York.

Bailey K D (1987) *Methods of Social Research,* 3rd edn. Macmillan, London.

Balfour S E (1989) Will I be in pain? Patients' and nurses' attitudes to pain after abdominal surgery. *Professional Nurse* 5(1), 28–33.

Beattie A (1987) Making a curriculum work. In Allan P and Jolley M (Eds) *The Curriculum in Nursing Education.* Chapman & Hall, London, pp. 15–34.

Bond M R (1984) *Pain: Its Nature, Analysis and Treatment.* Churchill Livingstone, Edinburgh.

Bondestam E, Hovgren K, Gaston Johansson F, Jern S and Herlitz J (1987) Pain assessment by patients and nurses in the early phase of acute myocardial infarction. *Journal of Advanced Nursing* 12(6), 677–82.

Boore J (1978) *Prescription for Recovery.* Royal College of Nursing, London.

Bourbonnais F (1981) Pain assessment: development of a tool for the nurse and the patient. *Journal of Advanced Nursing* 6(4), 277–82.

Broome A (1986) Strategies for relief. *Nursing Times* 82, 16 April, 43–4.

Cannon S (1989) Social research in stressful settings: difficulties for the sociologist studying the treatment of breast cancer. *Sociology of Health and Illness* 11(1), 62–77.

Carr E (1990a) A no-touch technique. *Nursing: The Journal of Clinical Practice, Education and Management* 4, 11 January, 9–11.

Carr E (1990b) Postoperative pain: patients' expectations and experiences. *Journal of Advanced Nursing* 15(1), 89–100.

Carr W and Kemmis S (1986) *Becoming Critical: Education, Knowledge and Action Research.* Falmer Press, London.

Child D (1986) *Psychology and the Teacher*. Holt, Rinehart & Winston, London.

Cohen L and Manion L (1980) *Research Methods in Education*. Croom Helm, London.

Cormack D F S (Ed.) (1984) *The Research Process in Nursing*. Blackwell Scientific, Oxford.

Davis P (1988) Changing nursing practice for more effective control of post operative pain through a staff initiated educational programme. *Nurse Education Today* 8(6), 325–31.

Davis P and Seers K (1991) Teaching nurses about managing pain. *Nursing Standard* 5, 18 September, 30–2.

Denzin N K (1989) *The Research Act: A Theoretical Introduction to Sociological Methods*. Prentice-Hall, Englewood Cliffs.

Duffy M E (1987) Methodological triangulation: a vehicle for merging quantitative and qualitative research methods. *Image: Journal of Nursing Scholarship* 19(3), 130–3.

Ewan C and White R (1984) *Teaching Nursing*. Chapman & Hall, London.

Gaston Johansson F and Asklund Gustafsson M (1985) A baseline study for the development of an instrument for the assessment of pain. *Journal of Advanced Nursing* 10(6), 539–46.

Geden E A, Lower M, Beattie S and Beck N (1989) Effects of music and imagery on physiologic and self-report of analogued labour pain. *Nursing Research* 38(1), 37–41.

Grace S (1990) Giving preoperative information – nursing opinion of, and methods currently practiced within one district general hospital. Unpublished dissertation, Buckinghamshire College of Higher Education.

Graffam S (1981) Congruence of nurse–patient expectations regarding nursing intervention in pain. *Nursing Leadership* 4(2), 12–15.

Graffam S (1990) Pain content in the curriculum – a survey. *Nurse Educator* 15(1), 20–3.

Hayward J (1975) *Information – A Prescription Against Pain*. Royal College of Nursing, London.

Holm K, Cohen F, Dudas S, Medema P G and Allen B L (1989) Effect of personal pain experience on pain assessment. *Image: Journal of Nursing Scholarship* 21(2), 72–5.

Holter I M and Schwartz-Barcott D (1993) Action research: what is it? How has it been used and how can it be used in nursing? *Journal of Advanced Nursing* 18, 298–304.

Hosking J and Welchew E (1985) *Postoperative Pain: Understanding Its Nature and How to Treat It*. Faber & Faber, London.

Hough A (1986) Handling the patient in pain. *Nursing Times* 82, 9 April, 28–31.

International Council of Nurses (1973) *Code for Nurses: Ethical Concepts Applied to Nursing*. ICN, Geneva.

Jacox A (1977) *Pain: A Source Book for Nurses and Other Health Professionals*. Little Brown, Boston.

Ketchin V Y (1989) Approaches to pain management. *Surgical Nurse* 2(2), 19–20, 22.

Kitson A (1988) Caring Standards. *Nursing Standard* 3, 5 November, 12–14.

Lockstone C (1982) It's what the patient says it is. *Nursing Mirror* 154, 17 February, Clinical Forum 2, i–xvi.

Long B C and Phipps W J (1984/85) *Essentials of Medical–Surgical Nursing.* Mosby, St Louis.

Madjar I (1985) Pain and the surgical patient: a cross-cultural perspective. *Australian Journal of Advanced Nursing* 2(2), 29–33.

Marks, R M and Sachar E J (1973) Under-treatment of medical inpatients with narcotic analgesics. *Annals of Internal Medicine* 78, 173–8.

McCaffery M (1980) Understanding your patient's pain. *Nursing 80* 10(9), 28–31.

McCaffery M (1983) *Nursing the Patient in Pain.* Faber & Faber, London.

McGuire D (1984) The measurement of clinical pain. *Nursing Research* 33(3), 152–6.

Miller A E (1979) Nurses' attitudes towards their patients. *Nursing Times* 15, 8 November, 1929–33.

Miller M A and Malcolm N S (1990) Critical thinking in the nursing curriculum. *Nursing and Health Care* 11(2), 67–73.

Murphy P A and Albers L L (1992) Evaluation of research studies part II: observational studies. *Journal of Nurse-Midwifery* 37(6), 411–13.

Nisbet J and Watt J (1980) *Case Study.* TRC-Rediguides, Oxford.

Oliver G (1989) Management and control of pain. *Primary Health Care* 7(1), 18–19.

Polit D and Hungler B (1985) *Nursing Research: Principles and Methods.* Lippincott, New York.

Pryn S (1992) *Staff Feedback on Analgesia Questionnaire.* Anaesthetic Department, Wycombe General Hospital. Internal Publication.

Quinn F M (1988) *The Principles and Practice of Nurse Education.* Chapman & Hall, London.

Raiman J (1986) Pain relief – a two-way process. *Nursing Times* 82, 9 April, 24–8.

Reid B (1991) Developing and documenting a qualitative methodology. *Journal of Advanced Nursing* 16, 544–51.

Rowntree D (1981) *Statistics Without Tears.* Penguin, Harmondsworth.

Roy C (1984) *Introduction to Nursing – An Adaptation Model.* Prentice-Hall, Englewood Cliffs.

Royal College of Nursing (1990) *The Dynamic Standard Setting System.* Royal College of Nursing, London.

Sandelowski M (1986) The problem of rigor in qualitative research. *Advances in Nursing Science* 8(3), 23–37.

Saxey S (1986) The nurse's response to postoperative pain. *Nursing: The Add-on Journal of Clinical Nursing* 3(10), 377–81.

Seers K (1987) Perceptions of pain. *Nursing Times* 83, 2 December, 37–9.

Sofaer B (1984) The effect of focused education for nursing teams on post-operative pain of patients. PhD thesis, University of Edinburgh, RCN Steinburg Collection.

Thomas B L (1991) Pain management for the elderly: alternative interventions (Part II). *AORN Journal* 53(1), 126–32.

Titlebaum H M (1988) Relaxation. *Holistic Nursing Practice* 2(3), 17–25.

Treece E W and Treece J W (1986) *Elements of Research in Nursing.* Mosby, St Louis.

Vines S W (1988) The therapeutics of guided imagery. *Holistic Nursing Practice* 2(3), 34–44.

Wainwright P (1990) Observation and the research process. *Nursing Standard* 4(43), 39–40.

Walding M F (1991) Pain, anxiety and powerlessness. *Journal of Advanced Nursing* 16(4), 388–97.

Walker R (1983) Three good reasons for not doing case studies in curriculum research. *Journal of Curriculum Studies* 15(2), 155–65.

Walker J M, Akinsanya J A, Davis B D and Marcer D (1989) The nursing management of pain in the community: a theoretical framework. *Journal of Advanced Nursing* 14(3), 240–7.

Watt-Watson J (1987) Nurses' knowledge of pain issues; a survey. *Journal of Pain and Symptom Management* 2(4), 207–11.

Webb C (1990) Partners in research. *Nursing Times* 86(32), 40–4.

Woodrow K (1972) Pain tolerance: differences according to age, sex and race. *Psychosomatic Medicine* 34(6), 548–56.

6

Readiness to learn?

Alison Goulbourne

Alison clearly captures in this chapter the different emotions and challenges that a novice researcher faces. In particular:

- *she reflects on her mistakes and offers clear strategies to overcome them. Clearly, correct use of a supervisor is one of these. The story around devising a research problem clearly shows a different approach to the other writers;*
- *the chapter also offers an excellent strategy for systematic cataloguing of literature so that there is no last-minute search for a remote reference;*
- *as part of the research design reliability and validity are explored;*
- *perhaps one of the most exciting aspects of this chapter is Alison's account of her journey to statistical proficiency. There is a wealth of learning in this account.*

Introduction

'Every man who rises above the common level has received two educations: the first from his teachers; the second, more personal and important, from himself'. (Gibbon, cited in Cooper, 1978)

This quotation sums up the topic and content of what I am trying to illustrate in this chapter. In 1992 I undertook an investigative study which rapidly grew beyond the realms necessary for a first degree. In fact, such was its scale that permission had to be granted to take into account its word limit!

Although I was beginning to become suspicious of its proportions approximately two-thirds of the way into the process, I was uncertain as to why this had actually occurred, or what I could do about it – if anything.

Writing about my personal experiences of doing research has helped me to make sense of these reasons. As Gibbon eloquently illustrates, some acknowledgement of my research achievement is attributable to my teachers, but mostly it was down to myself. Although this sounds a little arrogant I must stress that my level of enthusiasm landed me in hot water on more than one occasion. This chapter explains how this happened, the problems I subsequently incurred and how well (or otherwise) I handled them. In short it is a narrative of my developing role as a researcher.

Discerning readers involved in doing research for the first time – take heed. The end certainly justifies the means, but there are times when you seriously wonder. I now know that it is normal for every researcher, no matter how experienced, to feel this. I would go as far as to say that, as a normal aspect of the research process, it is the exception for researchers not to feel exasperated as well as exhilarated. Knowing this before hand may have made my venture into the realms of research less fretful.

Before I begin to describe these first-hand experiences, I would very much like to introduce myself as a 'researcher'. This will put into context how my learning became far more 'personal and important' (Gibbon) as a direct result of doing this research.

Myself as researcher

The title of this chapter reflects two things. First a summary of the research I completed in 1992:

> the extent to which pre-registration nursing students demonstrated *readiness* for self-directed learning, and the factors that influenced various degrees of readiness. (Goulbourne, 1992)

The study used quantitative and qualitative methods respectively, but for the purpose of this chapter I will only refer to the experiences encountered when choosing to use quantitative methods.

Secondly, just how ready was I to undertake an independent investigative study? At the time I genuinely believed that following a tenuous course of enquiry, called the 'research process', my data collection would not only be systematic and organized, but expose findings that would test and push back the boundaries of nursing knowledge. In short, the process of my study would resemble those documented in academically refereed journals – it would be polished, painless and unproblematic. I was about to learn a very important lesson.

I used Gibbon's quotation to open my dissertation as I felt it emphasized the idea that self-direction enhances meaningful learning. It does. My experiences testify to this fact. The extent of Gibbon's sentiments became personally apparent when the study was near completion as I understood how different the pragmatics of research were from the final product. This could only have been gleaned from first-hand experience.

This begs the question as to why am I bothering to write about this experience at all? If lessons can only be learned first hand, perhaps this exercise is just a little self-indulgent? Who exactly am I writing for? People may want to read about my ideas, but will they be really interested in why they have emerged?

Communicating understanding through writing is the articulation of academic theory. But is it possible to articulate academic theoretical principles about research through personal reflection? Despite the arguments that research must be objective and systematic for meaningful data to be reliable and valid (Lancaster, 1975; Goodwin and Goodwin, 1984; Stacey, 1988) the whole process of doing research is anything but objective or orderly. It is a messy process, that unravels the meanings behind why nurses do what they do.

In the research arena these essential differences between subjectivity of process and objectivity of product are fundamental for investigating the richness and complexity that epitomizes nursing knowledge. I shall try and illustrate my point.

The thought of graduating with a decent honours degree ensured effort was enough to make the experience academically worthwhile. However, as the study progressed, motivation became far more personal, and turned worthwhile effort into a tour de force. It was at the stage when my literature review was becoming problematic that I began to feel a tremendous sense of ownership of this assignment. Granted, this piece of work contributed a great deal to the final mark, but essentially it was still only just one of the many assignments that culminated in attaining my degree.

Only it wasn't! It was beyond the realms of a first class honours degree, but that was not really the point. Analysing the reasons as to why I did not heed my supervisor's advice as to this fact has led me to conclude that I was genuinely unable to act on it. My increasing motivation (and frustration) was reducing my capacity for listening to outside help. Guidance at the outset would no doubt have distinguished degree level boundaries, but the importance of this information would have become less as the study progressed.

As the research was assuming greater priority in my life, it was beginning to take on its own individuality, separate from the course. How could I remain an objective entity in my study when it was so essentially a part of me? It was awesome to think that my questions, to my knowledge, had never been thoroughly investigated before. Feelings and emotions swung between isolation, when things were not going my way, to exhilaration, when they were.

Several steps away from my research, I can now understand the reason for this change of attitude: I was no longer a student doing research for my degree, I was a researcher, a pioneer, hungry to find answers to questions I was initiating.

This developing identity as a researcher, and the personal experiences involved in this transitional process, are hardly discussed in research manuals and journals, yet it is such a pivotal aspect of the research process, it is almost taken for granted. I just wish someone had told me about it before I started. Even though it may have made no difference to how I approached and worked with the study at the time, it may have made a difference as to how I felt about myself then as a student, and now as a teacher supervising others experiencing their first taste of research.

Background to the study

Given that the research process is anything but logical, systematic or linear, it is not easy to identify a starting point. However, for the sake of clarity, I will attempt accurately to record events at a suitable juncture that suggests a start.

The starting point for any investigative study begins with a question. All I had to do was find out what burning questions I had. This is all part of the background to the study, and is as important an aspect of the process as any other. This was the first stage, the most important, and in many ways the hardest.

Much of the actual doing of research is refined in the thinking. Getting it right at the outset meant choosing the right subject which would not only sustain interest and motivation, but steer a course through a mire of data, deadlines and, at times, drudgery.

I deliberately set time aside systematically to reflect on what was important to me. A good deal of this reflection was preceded by late night conversations with my long suffering friends and husband. This reflective time would eventually lead to a review of available literature in order to focus my area of study. This was accomplished during a holiday.

Perhaps including time for course work during a holiday was indication enough as to the project's potency – I had not done this before, or since. However, before this stage had been reached I simply asked myself what it was about nursing education that concerned me most. I was ready to write a checklist, but the answer came quickly.

As a student nurse teacher, I was becoming more aware that teaching and learning could be mutually exclusive. In other words, students would learn despite the teaching they received, rather than because of it. This educational dichotomy had obvious implications for how I felt about my newfound role. I realized that in order to tackle the problem I first had to understand it.

I realized the dynamics between teaching and learning were far more complex than I first supposed. For a start, there were apparently two major theoretical approaches to educating others: 'pedagogy', the teaching of children, and 'andragogy', the teaching of adults (Knowles, 1973, 1978).

According to Knowles (1973, 1978), each approach necessitated a different teaching style. This style depended on the individual's level of maturity, maturity being more than an assumed biological age, but the individual's ability critically to contextualize past and present experiences. As children have fewer life experiences, skills and knowledge to evaluate given situations they are less 'mature'. Therefore, the overall approach to teaching children is more explanatory in style than discursive.

Age is a factor which promotes maturity, simply because of the time available to accumulate a wealth of knowledge and experience. Sharing these experiences with others is paramount for developing skills appropriate to adult learning theory. Reflecting on past situations to help make sense of the present enables critical thinking and so maturity of intellect (Brookfield, 1988). Discursive styles of teaching, therefore, promote adult learning behaviours.

This mode of acquiring maturity in learning does not automatically preclude children. A child may have amassed more experiences in a relatively short period of time than some adults, but their level of cognisance does not enable experiences to be contextually evaluated and transformed into personal and meaningful learning. The knowledge any student brings to a learning situation initiates a dynamic process of learning between student and teacher; the more 'mature' or 'adult' the student, the more involved they ought to be in their own education (Bruner, 1966; Grow, 1991).

Valuing the experiences each student brings to any learning situation is pivotal to a theory of andragogy. Sharing knowledge which has personal relevance for students is enhanced by teaching styles that permit reflection and analysis of these individual experiences. In short, adult education enhances the 'personal' in learning: it is a learning process driven by students, but navigated by teachers.

Refining the research area

Now that a problem area was beginning to emerge, it needed to be developed and refined in order to shape a researchable question.

Defining a research question involves a considerable degree of overlap in research stages, namely literature search and review. Searching the literature relevant to an emerging concern or hunch was an unsystematic process that helped me finally to decide the what, as well as the how, of my research. I was fortunate that this stage of the process turned out to be so fruitful: deriving a focus from a literature search can be expected, but finding the method was a bonus.

Now that I understood the essential differences in educational ideologies, it was becoming clearer why teaching did not always precede learning – the students were adult learners. Teaching styles were often inappropriate for the educational stage of these mature students. On reflection, this should not have been such a surprise for, as studies had already shown, nurses are adults by the very nature of what they do in practice (Heath,

1979; Hollingworth, 1980; Sweeney, 1986; Brookfield, 1988; Richardson, 1988; Burnard, 1990). The complexity of practical situations means that nurses have to be able to think on their feet. Being professional implies nurses are self-motivated, independent learners, who are creative in finding answers to guide their practice.

Self-directed learning appeared to complement this creative process of thinking, as it gave students the necessary skills in finding solutions to problems. This process was also synonymous with the ability to make decisions basic to delivering individualized care.

This notion of 'self-directed learning' was a confusing educational term, but I understood it to mean educational freedom to select the content and methods of learning. As a nursing educationalist, it was a behaviour I ought to be encouraging in the students.

This was all well and good, but my experiences with the students revealed that enthusiasm for self-directed learning was more apparent among the teaching staff than among the students. This was especially the case the more senior the students became. If educational rhetoric was to be believed, the third year students I taught should have been far more independent and confident in their learning than the second and first years. However, I felt the opposite to be true.

My initial literature search showed my assumptions were not new. O'Kell's (1988) small study revealed that self-directed learning among undergraduate students did actually reduce with each successive year of training and, what was more, there was a method of testing it. A closer inspection of the data revealed inconsistencies in statistical analysis. Undaunted that O'Kell's findings were no longer valid, I was especially excited to find a study that parallelled my own interests and so provided a focus for my own study, while at the same time proposed a viable methodology.

Replication of the study was inappropriate for two reasons: the methodological inconsistencies and the additional, more professionally pertinent question I was subsequently asking – does pre-registered nursing students' motivation for self-directed learning behaviour reduce with seniority? This I could test using a pre-validated questionnaire that measured readiness for self-directed learning (Guglielmino, 1977). Also, how could I, as a teacher, help foster this learning behaviour? This meant subsequently interviewing selected students to discover factors that affected self-directed learning behaviour.

Considerations at this stage

Even though I was aware that my dissertation module was still six months away, it took all this available time before my research question was refined and the methodology identified. Although the area of concern was clear, there was scope for flexibility of ideas and specificity in direction. This additional information and refinement I needed to obtain from a literature search. If my ideas for research had been definite, the initial literature search would not have been as fruitful as it was, as searching for answers to questions that have not as yet been addressed is a frustrating and unnecessarily time-consuming process.

As it was, I remember feeling distinctly anxious that this aspect of the research process was taking too long and I needed to move on. This anxiety was perpetuated by the conviction that little was being accomplished, as nothing concrete had been committed to paper.

It is highly unlikely that the potential nurse researcher will suddenly decide on an area to focus a research study and so, in retrospect, the accomplishments during this preparatory stage were not insignificant. This achievement reflected the amount of valuable time and effort given to the first formal stage of the process – the planning.

The important lessons I learned at this stage were:

- Do not underestimate the importance of this aspect of research activity; it needs plenty of time for adequate clarification of thoughts. Thorough preparation will save time later.
- Flexibility in identifying an area of research will ensure the final chosen research question is both topical and personally relevant.

Refining the research question

Purpose, feasibility and definitions

Purpose

Initial searching of the literature had enabled a clear focus for both the topic and research methods. What I needed to do next was transform abstract ideas into a recognizable, understandable research title that clearly expressed research methodology and purpose. This was no mean feat!

The purpose of research reflects the goal, or justifies why the study is being conducted in the first place. Initial draft statements of my study did not justify a research purpose.

Even if Guglielmino's 'Self-Directed Learning Readiness Scale' (S.D.L.R.S., 1977) reliably validated assumptions that differences in readiness for self-directed learning existed among students at various stages of training – so what? Who was the main beneficiary of this evidence, myself as teacher, or the students themselves? As I needed a selection of willing participants to sample, the ultimate beneficiaries must be the students; any personal gain was a bonus.

Theoretical rhetoric expounded notions that self-directed learners were motivated, had a better understanding, were more self-fulfilled and improved the quality of education overall (Jones, 1981; Brockett, 1985;

Sweeney, 1986; Burnard, 1989). Understanding how to engender self-directed learning would benefit the recipients of nursing care, the students them-selves and the quality of my own teaching. The purpose of the research would be clearly articulated in this second part of the study.

However, I first needed to establish if nurses were self-directed in their learning, and, if so, did increasing seniority make any difference? The title of the study therefore read:

> Is there a relationship between the readiness for self-direction in learning, and increasing student seniority? An exploratory study identifying factors affecting readiness for self-directed learning between first, second and third year regis-tered general nursing students, in one college of nursing.

Feasibility

The clarity of purpose in the title helps determine the feasibility of the study; for example, constraints on time, finance and/or resources. As a finishing time had already been decided by course structure, the study had to be manageable, both in terms of its subject matter, access to the student groups and methodology.

However, considering appropriate methods involves not only the opera-tional feasibility, but also a mastery of data analysis; this had not as yet crossed my mind. My dearth in research knowledge and skills had consequences for appreciating that feasibility also entailed researcher expertise.

Considerations at this stage

I was relatively certain that the chosen problem was within my capabilities to investigate. I could access my targeted student population, and, although Guglielmino's 'Self-Directed Learning Readiness Scale' still needed to be procured, these questionnaires could be easily issued to first, second and third year students. However, I clearly did not have the know-how to perform quantitative analysis, but at this stage I was unaware what exactly this entailed. Consequently, I did not make any enquiries as to where, how or even if expert advice could be readily accessed. I was innocent of the fact that this lack of preparation and supervision would culminate in the study being almost abandoned much later on.

Although I subsequently feel advice at this stage could have been more apparent, I could have avoided this mistake if:

- I had discussed with my supervisor this aspect of the process, as I had all others.
- I appreciated that the naming of a study implies a good deal more than initially supposed.

Definitions

Nursing has many commonly used vague terms which are poorly defined and prone to bewilder the uninitiated as to their meaning and use; for example, the term 'patient' may refer to a child, adult or person with psychological or physical problems. How these concepts are defined differs, depending on their contextual use and terms of reference.

The use of unambiguous terms in nursing literature minimizes the chance of readers placing personal interpretation on central concepts. This is obligatory in the field of research, as clearly operationally defined terms will help the researcher decide which methods of data collection are more appropriate. This ensures validity of data and hopefully reliability of findings that can be confidently utilized to inform practice.

My own research title had three generic concepts that needed specific clarification:

Student group

This term was easy to define as students could be identified as pre-registered general nursing students on a 146 week training course. The level of seniority referred to their respective year of training.

The remaining two concepts were not so easy to clarify and operationalize.

Self-directed learning

A literature review soon revealed that a coherent, uniform acceptance of what constituted self-directed learning did not exist.

Opinion differed depending on whether it was perceived as an attitude of mind or a behavioural trait. For example, O'Kell (1988), Oddi (1986) and Iwasiw (1987) described this mode of learning as a 'process' while Hamilton and Gregor (1986) and Wiley (1983) perceived it to be an observable activity, implying that self-direction is a behaviour. Others (Sweeney, 1986; Grow, 1991) saw self-direction as an individual quality, an attitude that precedes behavioural indicators which suggests personal responsibility and autonomy for learning. These two attributes, attitude and behaviour, were paramount in operationalizing definitions of both self-directed learning and readiness.

I understood self-directed learning to be essentially a mental attitude which is exhibited in recognizable behavioural characteristics which were validated by independent corroborative studies (Knowles, 1973; Guglielmino, 1977) (Figure 6.1).

The ability to be a self-directed learner was not innate. Preliminary factors had to be gradually taken on board before a student was perceived as being essentially adult in their learning. As stated before, self-direction

FACTOR – (Guglielmino, 1977) DIMENSIONS OF MATURITY – (Knowles, 1973)

FACTOR – (Guglielmino, 1977)	DIMENSIONS OF MATURITY – (Knowles, 1973)
1. Self Concept as an effective learner	Autonomy, activity, enlightenment, large abilities, many responsibilities, deep concerns, broad interests, integrated self-identify, self-acceptance
2. Openness to learning opportunities	Large abilities, tolerance for ambiguity
3. Initiative and independence in learning	Autonomy, activity, large abilities, focus on principles, reality, rationality
4. Acceptance of responsibility for one's own learning	Autonomy, objectivity, integrated self-identity, self-identify
5. Love of learning	Enlightenment, many responsibilities, broad interests, deep concerns, tolerance for ambiguity
6. Creativity	Enlightenment, broad interests, deep concerns, integrated self-identity, tolerance for ambiguity
7. Ability to use problem-solving skills and basic study skills	Activity, autonomy, objectivity, large abilities, focus on principles, rationality reality
8. Positive orientation to the future	Large abilities, many responsibilities, broad interests, altruism, self-acceptance, integrated self-identity, deep concerns

Figure 6.1 Critical dimensions of maturity

was only the outward behaviour that indicated something far more significant, yet so abstract in nature it was becoming more difficult to define, not to mention measure. Thanks to even more educational rhetoric, this nebulous term became clearer.

Depending on an individual's orientation to learning at a given time, the gradual process of self-directed learning behaviour meant incorporating personal knowledge into practical experience. This gradual process was achieved by understanding the relevance and use of core skills, central for self-directed learning ability. These skills were essentially dependent on the ability of the teacher effectively to elucidate and develop the pragmatic use of academic theory in students. For example, mastering skills of reflection and analysis would enable a growing awareness of self to accurately assess personal strengths and weaknesses. A consistent level of maturity would then be retained and developed with or without the teacher's assistance.

In short these skills and abilities enhanced critical thinking processes (Brookfield, 1988). The ability to think critically distinguished a learner as mature, responsible and therefore adult, capable of taking on a vast array of practical experiences, pertinent to everyday work.

The term 'critical thinking' needed clarification in itself, but at this stage it was important not to become side-tracked; I was on a roll!

What was fascinating was the emerging evidence that suggested certain predisposing factors did affect self-directed learning. Top of the list was the teacher!

Knowles (1973), cited by Conti (1985), suggested that the teacher was the most important factor influencing the nature of the learning climate. Through their teaching style feelings were conveyed regarding relationships with students. Teaching style being yet another ambiguous term needed clarification:

> Our use of style refers to a pervasive quality in the *behaviour* of an individual, a quality that persists even though the content may change . . . Style is not to be confused with method. (Fischer and Fischer, 1979, p. 14)

Likewise, Kuchinskas (1979) found no matter what the content being taught, the teacher's behaviour was the overwhelming factor that affected everyone. There appeared to be a positive correlation between teaching style and degree of self-direction in students.

Iwasiw (1987) and Grow (1991) saw it was the teacher's responsibility to ensure the smooth transition from dependent to independent learner. If dependency and helplessness could be learned, then so could self-direction.

As Brookfield (1988) had already attested, the acceptance for self-directed learning is relative to the student's expectations and learning capabilities at a given moment. Beginning students needed more guidance and supervision; as the learner's knowledge base increases, then the educational processes should be more student-centred. Self-direction is a facilitated process of learning: a balance between learning capabilities and teaching demands.

Readiness

Observing self-directed learning behaviour in students at various stages in training was my objective for the first part of the study. A concept analysis had revealed that self-direction was an outward behaviour that indicated something far more important – the student's state of learning readiness.

> Readiness as a developmental task, associated with moving from one stage of development to another. (Knowles, 1978, p. 237)

The literature had already stipulated that self-directed learning was not an innate feature in students, but a process which needed to be learned. Depending upon life's experiences at a given moment, students could only ever be ready to pursue an aspect of self-direction in their learning, as total learning autonomy assumed complete independence.

Readiness proposes more than curiosity and a willingness to learn but demonstrates that one can also master self-directed behaviour. A current level of readiness for self-directed learning is subject to change, as its existence is relative to time and situation.

Readiness, then, is an attitude of mind which encompasses motivation and capability for the manifestation of self-directed learning behaviour.

Considerations at this stage

Operationalizing concepts is relatively straightforward if the definitions have universal meanings, or are fairly concrete in their use. 'Self-directed learning' was neither universal or concrete. Hunting for a definition that was useable was difficult, as interpretation of the meaning must be consistent throughout the study. 'Readiness', although more abstract, was an easier term to define, as its meanings were generic. For this same reason, 'student' was also easy to define and interpret.

Although a difficult process, operationalizing terms is fundamental for interpreting a particular research approach and design of study. Reasons for this will become apparent when this stage of the process is considered. Difficult or not, the developing outline of the study was guiding me further into a mire of literature, which was rapidly becoming overwhelming.

There is no discernible point at which searching the literature becomes a rigorous review. For me it occurred when I recognized the symptom of information overload – I was drowning in a plethora of data. I needed a systematic and organized approach to analyse my literature.

The literature review

Evaluating relevant literature is a central part of the research process and accounts for a large percentage of the total effort involved.

I am aware that the way I have chosen to sequence the research process for this chapter would appear to indicate that, as yet, no discernible literature review had been conducted. If that were so, then very little progress would have been made.

As mentioned earlier, potential confusion arises because searching and reviewing the literature are closely related aspects of the research process, but their different functions require different skills. Reviewing the literature necessitates critical evaluation of reports, articles abstracts and any other forms of publication that systematically probe the research question obtained as a result of a search.

My ultimate aim from the literature review was to combine hunches with a more formal and systematic analysis of previous studies. However, as a review should reflect depth and breadth of analysis pertinent to the question, it was important to me to have a clear research title to ensure analysis was relevant to the question. This helped in structuring the review. It would have been quite possible to spend an inordinate amount of precious time stuck at this stage of the process. I had to be sensible and put a self-imposed moratorium on fact-gathering before I either blew up the photocopier or drowned in a mountain of articles.

Cataloguing all articles alphabetically, with a brief summary of what the item entailed, was invaluable when it came to writing a structured coherent review, and referencing my sources. I used two different coloured index cards. One colour was used to catalogue literature that had immediate relevance on my subject matter. The other cards listed studies or discussion papers that related in some way to my project, but had no direct bearing, for instance, research designs for measuring effective teaching methods, or learning styles and occupational choices of nurses. In this way I allowed myself to be side-tracked but could keep the field in which I was searching the literature within limits.

Articles themselves were filed under main headings that had direct relevance to the study, for example, nurse education, teaching methods, research methods, nurses as learners, educational theory, etc. In this way, extraneous papers that did not appear to fit with the general topic could be kept separate.

Discarding obscure material would have been disastrous, not only for my subsequent compilation of references, but for ensuring breadth as well as depth of literary analysis. I probably utilized 75 per cent of what I amassed. If I had not secured a title to keep me focused, I might still be collecting information now, or at the very least, my review would have rapidly become unmanageable. As it was, anything with 'self-direction' or similar permeations in the heading was automatically grabbed from library shelves. Hence I amassed a great deal more information than I either needed, or could possibly use. However, it was all useful in the long run, so I was pleased nothing was pitched on impulse.

When it came to writing up various stages of the study, I was glad that these pain-staking methods of cataloguing information were implemented. My systematic approach to filing, listing, summarizing and indexing paid off as I never once lost that vital article budding literalists need to stem writer's block.

I would have benefited from using a plan at the outset, as this would have acted as a guiding framework for the production of my review. Benton and Cormack (1991) suggest one such guiding framework (Figure 6.2). Findings can then be related to the overall planned structure. This would have saved an inestimable amount of time.

I very much intended to keep my review focused on the central issues concerned: examining evidence that suggested a relationship existed between readiness for self-direction in learning and student seniority, and the factors that affected a student's self-directed learning ability. I was not wanting to discover if the relationship was causal; that would be ascertained when factors that affected readiness for self-directed learning were examined.

For this reason, the status of nurses' academic profile was considered in relation to other professionals, such as lawyers and teachers. These professions were chosen as their acquisition of knowledge was through educational processes rather than training.

Theoretical assumptions regarding preferred learning styles nurses adopted both historically and contemporarily were reviewed, as well as

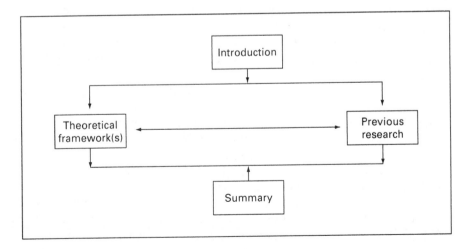

Figure 6.2 Literature review outline

known factors that influence a student's readiness for self-direction. These factors eventually formed the basis for an interview schedule and included:

- the nature of the learning climate;
- teachers' attitudes and styles;
- student participation in teaching-learning processes;
- teaching methods (namely the lecture);
- previous learning experiences;
- individual learning styles.

Although an illuminating aspect of the study, it bears little relevance to the purpose of this chapter, as this entailed the use of qualitative methods and analysis.

A comprehensive review of information also led to incorporating other aspects of the study. A large proportion of the review helped establish conceptual clarity, justification of methods and analysis of Guglielmino's (1977) own research and the resulting S.D.L.R.S.

All these different perspectives made this stage of the research process arduous. The more information I gathered, the more perplexing the initial problem became. I was not sure what to discard, what to keep or what to do with it all, if I decided to keep it.

There was a good deal of overlap, repetition and general disorganization that I was not able to rectify until the study was nearly completed. Textbooks told me that a well organized review should clearly identify various theoretical perspectives, identify strengths and weaknesses of each and compare similarities and differences (Burns and Grove, 1987; Chinn and Kramer, 1991; Polgar and Cormack, 1991; Thomas, 1991). Gaps in knowledge could then be easily identified, and I could form a clear rationale for conducting my study and developing future research. It was easier to identify gaps in my memory than nursing knowledge, as I was often distracted by studies that appeared to tackle the debate but turned out to be irrelevant. This meant that there were times I could not remember what it was I was supposed to be looking for, or why I needed particular information.

I am sure some experienced researchers may point to the fact that my downfall was the lack of initial planning. However, I only understood the nature of the problem I was researching once I had completed my analysis. My own findings meant I could ruthlessly decide what was relevant in the review, and what was extraneous and confusing.

Perhaps I cheated, but I feel in my heart that any research that involves studying the nature of people means researchers cannot afford to be rigorously systematic in their approach for fear of losing vital information in the process. As it was, I feel the review was objective and relevant to the problem I had chosen to investigate, and criticism was balanced and supportive of factual material and appropriate evidence. The following is a summary of my findings.

Relevant literary findings

Nurses were undoubtedly adult in their approach to learning (Clarke and Dickenson, 1976, Emblen and Gray, 1990) and so displayed self-directed learning characteristics. Evidence to show whether self-direction increases or decreases through basic nurse training was conflicting and so needed further investigation. My assumptions were well founded and justified the initial focus of the study: to ascertain if a relationship exists between readiness for self-directed learning and student seniority, readiness being a combination of motivation and abilities (Hersey and Blanchard, cited in Grow, 1991).

Considerations at this stage

- A sense of disorderliness and chaos is not unusual. I found it imperative to celebrate and commiserate with fellow students. This was my greatest source of reassurance.
- A plan of appropriate information generated from an already constructed research title would have prevented a growing sense of unease and saved a good deal of time.
- Do not be tempted to keep collecting articles. There will always be more data, but if the new information does not clearly contribute to the discussion, the review has come full circle.
- Systematic cataloguing is vital if references are not to be lost later.
- Although intensive at the start, the review of the literature is continuous throughout all the various stages of the process, and has particular relevance for the latter part of the study – namely the discussion and analysis.

Research design and methods

Design

Design of the overall research approach is different from the means of how data is collected. Thus, the data collection method(s) are a part of the research design.

Decisions regarding research design precede selection of data collection methods. The selection of design is based on grounds of what is best suited to answer the research question: the most suitable methods of data collection are then selected.

Readiness for self-direction, for the benefit of this study, had been described as an attitude that predisposes self-directed learning behaviour. These characteristics are readily accepted and recognized as being attributes of a mature learner (Figure 6.1).

Knowledge regarding readiness could be systematically classified and organized through sensory interpretation. Readiness for self-directed learning is an empirical phenomena, whereby pertinent facts are observed, described and validated, in order to measure differences in behaviour between first, second and third-year student nurses.

According to Chinn and Kramer (1991), empirical knowledge has three aspects: the 'symbolizing dimension' *describing* what is observed; the 'understanding dimension' *explaining* what is observed; and the 'creating dimension' *predicting* the future occurrence of what is observed.

Measuring readiness for self-directed learning for this study only involved two of these three aspects – 'symbolizing' and 'understanding'. The 'creating' dimension of empirics that predicts and hypothesizes outcomes was not a facet of the study's design, as research had demonstrated that characteristics precipitating self-directed learning behaviour were relative and subject to the individual's developing maturity. Any attempt to manipulate or control these factors would have been impossible. For this reason, the approach used was not truly experimental in design but quasi-experimental (Burns and Grove, 1987; Cohen and Manion, 1989).

> Quantitative researchers collect facts and study the relationship of one set of facts to another. They measure, using scientific techniques that are likely to produce quantified and, if possible, generalisable conclusions. (Bell, 1987, p. 4)

As findings of quasi-experimental research cannot be generalized, results would not be as powerful as true experimental research.

If new meanings of reality are discovered through quasi-experimental processes that measure and recount how often phenomena occur, the researcher is using a descriptive approach in their research design (Marriner, 1980). Therefore, the research approach was quantitative; the design descriptive, quasi-experimental.

Methods

Using Guglielmino's questionnaire type S.D.L.R.S. (1977) I would measure differences in readiness for self-directed learning between first, second and third-year student nurses.

This measurement addressed the 'symbolic' and 'understanding' aspects of empirics. For example, by using a questionnaire method, symbolic interpretation of another's maturity was measured objectively through recognized characteristics that described self-directed learning behaviour in student nurses. Explanation of what was observed was then executed through the measurement of different self-directed readiness scores between successive years of training.

Reliability and validity

Conceptual definitions were operationalized to suit a given quantitative research design and chosen survey method. However, in order to substantiate the study's scientific merit I needed to demonstrate more than just face validity.

Instruments used for the collection of data must be tested for reliability and construct validity.

Reliability refers to accuracy and consistency of the tool, while construct validity is concerned with the instrument's ability to measure what it is supposed to measure (Burns and Grove, 1987; Heyes *et al.*, 1988; Cormack, 1991). Competent practitioners would not try to measure blood pressure using a thermometer. Although ensuring validity and reliability of methods is less problematic with quantitative than qualitative studies, it is no less important. Any study, no matter what approach, is measured by the degree of merit awarded to these two facets of investigation processes: reliability and validity.

This meant delving deeper into the literature. I was beginning to wonder when the review stage would finally be finished!

The process of developing construct validity for an instrument often requires years of scientific work (Heyes *et al.*, 1988; Polgar and Thomas, 1991). It was over 16 years since Lucy Guglielmino devised her scale as part of her doctoral research.

Since its development, the scale's reliability and validity had been repeatedly tested through its continual application in various studies (Torrance and Mourad, 1978; Savoie, 1980; Skaggs, 1981; Katherein, 1982; Box, 1983; Long and Agyekum, 1984, Crook, 1985).

To understand what others had written regarding Guglielmino's original work, I needed to grapple with statistical language. Statistical language is so specialized it appears to be inaccessible to inexperienced researchers. I could have been easily persuaded to look the other way if I did not have a statistics book which translated unintelligible jargon into discernible English. The book which helped me steer a clear course through this potentially incomprehensible field was Heyes *et al.* (1988). This gives basic information, relevant to analysing descriptive statistics. For subsequent analysis more complex text had to be waded through (Siegel and Castellan, 1988; Polgar and Thomas, 1991).

The S.D.L.R.S. was designed to assess the extent to which an individual perceives themselves to possess self-directed learning characteristics. The instrument was devised using a three-round Delphi Survey: a consultative data collecting method that gradually accumulates ideas and judgements from a group of perceived experts (Burns and Grove, 1987).

A consensus of opinion revealed that distinguishing self-directed learning behaviours could be catalogued as a 58 item, five-point Likert Scale: 'almost never true of me: I hardly ever feel this way', to 'almost always true of me: there are very few times when I don't feel this way'.

Values are placed on each score, 1 being negative and 5 positive (for the majority of responses).

Understanding general principles of questionnaire construction was manageable. Problems began to materialize when I began to examine the instrument's internal consistency.

Each item used on a questionnaire should relate to the general research question in some purposeful and unique way. There are statistical tests which are specifically designed to analyse consistency of purpose (item homogeneity), while at the same time examine inter-correlational relationships or the degree of relationship between two variables (Heyes *et al.*, 1988). For example, a dependent variable 'temperature' would correlate positively to the independent variable 'pyrexia' – if one is high, so is the other. Conversely, 'peripheral perfusion' would have a negative correlation with 'pyrexia'; one would decrease as the other increases. In statistical terms, this is known as the correlation coefficient (Burns and Grove, 1987; Heyes *et al.*, 1988).

A Cronbachs alpha is one such test that measures aspects of internal consistency or item homogeneity and correlational coefficient. The nearer to 0 the coefficient, the better the correlation. A coefficient above 0.8 suggests a good degree of homogeneity, and so relevance, consistency and validity; a value above 0.6 represents an acceptable degree of homogeneity; 0 indicates complete coalition (Heyes *et al.*, 1988). The S.D.L.R.S had a Cronbachs alpha of 0.87, and so demonstrated a good degree of construct validity.

Although Heyes *et al.* (1988) was a useful reference during this time, its utility was limited. Often statistical terms have no meaning that can be explained; understandings are derived from their contextual use. For example, just as the meanings behind the terms 'weather' or 'pain' are derived from their relationship with other words or phrases used in a given sentence, so is the case with a good deal of statistical language. Interpretations for some terms such as Chronbachs alpha do not exist outside the word itself – it assumes its own definition. Understanding often depends on personal interpretation and contiguous use.

Considerations at this stage

Although all this sounds complicated, justifying design and methodology to myself was relatively easy. Interpreting complex theories to justify a particular pragmatic approach necessitated clear understanding and articulation of concepts. It was now I really appreciated the time and effort spent on that particular aspect of the process. Thorough deconstruction of terms meant abstract definitions of readiness and self-direction were sufficiently operationalized to enable a quantitative investigative approach.

Turning intangible concepts into concrete terms is necessary for investigating empirical phenomena, but this may alter definitions and meanings in the process. I was confident that this had not been the case. I believed that I could progress, safe in the knowledge that the study had 'face validity' – it looked like it would do what it was supposed to do.

Ethical considerations

Confidentiality and anonymity

The planning stage was nearly completed. I was anxious to collect my data. Before I did so, it was important that I discussed with my supervisor all aspects of my intended methodological technique to reassure myself that in principle my research appeared sound. A well thought-out research strategy will reduce the chance of causing unintended harm or distress to people involved. An unbiased critique of my research plan would highlight erroneous aspects that I could have overlooked.

The literature search and review had enabled a convincing research question to be constructed that had face validity. My choice of research design and use of a measurement tool demonstrated construct validity and therefore could be justified. My research did have the potential to advance educational knowledge as my purpose was now clear. All that remained was the underlying ethical considerations implicit in the pragmatics of research methods. This included aspects of confidentiality and anonymity.

It was the objective observations of my supervisor that helped unravel a potentially knotty problem that could have caused anxiety to students at a later date. This was in relation to students whose scores demonstrated their inability to be self-directed.

Each questionnaire would be coded to indicate student group only. A slip of paper attached to each questionnaire had a corresponding code number. Should students wish to be contacted for subsequent interviewing, they were asked to return the signed slip with their questionnaires. Students not wanting to be interviewed could not be individually identified. Anonymity was secured; confidentiality would be addressed when interviews were processed.

Individual S.D.L.R.S. scores would not be known by the students unless specifically requested. The interviews could be used as an opportunity for personal development, and the student would be encouraged to continue discussion with their academic tutor. The risk to an individual's self-esteem would therefore be minimized. As it happened, this was never an issue, as the results of the analysis and limitations of the study will reveal.

A letter outlining the research proposal was drafted to the ethics committee of the college. Permission was granted, and I was ready to pilot my study.

The phase of the research process that addresses ethical considerations of a study is paramount. Therefore, the importance of supervision cannot be stressed enough, especially when people are the focus of the study. The supervisor must not only be familiar with the subject under scrutiny, but have had first-hand experience with research in order to secure a quality product. Anything less does a disservice to the researcher, the data produced and, most importantly, the people concerned.

As a student researcher, it is extremely difficult to foresee various ethical implications behind implementing research that directly involves people. Experience dealing with this sensitive arena is vital for identifying areas that could inadvertently traumatize and distress the people willing to take part.

The fact that this aspect of the research process was as straightforward as it appears to be on paper was testimony to the quality of supervision I received. My supervisor's expertise meant that potential problems were readily highlighted and addressed. The potentially perturbing areas I have described could not have been identified by myself, as I had limited educational and research experience. Even if I had been able to identify these potential problems for students with low scores, devising a strategy that adequately dealt with this would have been beyond my capabilities at the time.

My supervisor enabled a proactive approach when implementing the study. Hence, problems that subsequently arose were not ethical in origin, and could certainly not be attributed to my supervisor.

Piloting the method

I wanted to pilot the S.D.L.R.S to determine its practical efficacy for myself and students. For the students' benefit I needed to address the questionnaire's utility, by ascertaining timing and understanding. For myself, I needed to determine that the responses were clear and I could score accordingly.

Six students volunteered to be piloted, two first, two second and two third years. No students were taken from the actual research sample.

It took all six students no longer than 15 minutes to complete all 58 items. However, all six found the response options confusing, especially where this related to negatively scored items, for example, 'If I don't learn its not my fault' or 'I'll be glad when I'm finished learning'.

Guglielmino included these negatively phrased items to reduce response set, but students confessed to misreading the questions completely. This confusion would have skewed the results dramatically if the S.D.L.R.S. had not been piloted. Students reversed their questionnaire responses once they had been queried.

Likewise, all six students thought the qualifying statement in the response options – 'Almost always true of me: There are very few times when I don't think this way' – unnecessary and confusing, especially where this referred to the negatively phrased items.

These findings were unsettling, as the scale's reliability appeared to be dubious. This needed to be addressed by modifying the response options and omitting the qualifying statement as per the students' recommendations. I now needed to re-test the scale's reliability.

The students were issued the modified scales on two separate occasions.

Each time their scores were compared with their original S.D.L.R.S. scores (Table 6.1).

A positive correlation in post-test–retest scores are much higher than between original scale and post-test scores. Therefore the modified scale was reliable.

Although my heart sank when incongruities in the scale emerged, this initial experience with statistics was good preparation for what was to come. This simple exercise revealed how illuminating statistics could be, and boosted my confidence in the process.

Data analysis and statistics

Background and introduction to terms

This portion of the chapter discusses the analysis of quantitative data. Donnan (1991) states that 'good statistics start with good design' (p. 261) as a well designed study provides useful results and conclusions.

This is true no matter what research approach is adopted, but especially so when considering statistical analysis.

There are basically two approaches to analysing quantitative data, and the choice depends on the initial purpose of the study.

Descriptive statistics reduce the complexity of the world, and summarize the essence of situations by comparing differences in type, meaning and use of averages: for example, the 'mean' arithmetic average, the most commonly recurring number or 'mode', and the identifiable middle score in a series of ranked numbers or 'median' (Heyes *et al.*, 1988).

By examining the range or distribution of scores around the mean average, descriptive statistics can also display differences and relationships within a group. This measurement of 'standard deviation' (SD) is more useful than just an analysis of differences in average, as it takes into account all the scores and their relationship to the average number. This gives a far better description of a group overall, rather than looking at just one section (Heyes *et al.*, 1988; Donnan, 1991).

Table 6.1 Test–retest score correlation

Student Year	Original Scale	Post-test	Difference	Retest	Difference
1st	207	227	20	235	8
1st	201	214	13	225	11
2nd	215	230	15	233	3
2nd	238	248	10	248	0
3rd	219	262	43	255	7
3rd	169	193	24	197	4

Inferential statistics make future predictions based on information already obtained about a population; for example, the incidence of heart disease, child birth, or exam success rate. Inferential statistics make judgements and test hypotheses based on the reliability of past results. The larger the population, the less likely results have occurred by chance, and would probably be exactly the same should the experiment be repeated. In other words the results are significant and expressed in terms of percentages or P values as depicted in Table 6.2 (Heyes *et al.*, 1988; Donnan 1991).

The most common level of significance is 5 per cent (Hardy *et al.*, 1988). This means that if P is 5 per cent (0.05) or smaller, the result is significant, and will probably reoccur if the test is repeated. Inferential statistics are far more powerful than descriptive (Burns and Grove, 1987; Donnan, 1991; Thomas, 1991), but need large numbers to sample to ensure significance of results (Heyes *et al.*, 1988).

This background information can be found in any basic statistics textbook, but the reader has to know what it is that statistics can do in order to refer to the correct passage in the book!

Descriptive statistics did not yield the answers I was looking for, and so I stumbled accidentally and totally unaided into the realm of inferential statistics. At the time, I was unaware of these differences in quantitative data analysis. Had I known before hand, it would have been clear what the various stages of analysis were, and why I was doing what I was. What did happen occurred by good fortune rather than planning. The following is an account of how my learning curve rapidly soared as competent effort turned into chaos.

Using descriptive statistics

Questionnaires were distributed to three independent groups – first, second and third years. My relationship with the second and third years was good enough to secure good sized groups to sample. I was not so confident about the first years' willingness to participate as we had not met.

The total student population (n) I targeted numbered 105. Returned and

Table 6.2 Probability values

Probability in percentage (%)	Equivalent probability on the 0 to 1 scale
100	0.1
50	0.5
10	0.1
5	0.05
1	0.01

(Heyes *et al.*, 1986)

usable questionnaires numbered 62 per cent, which was very promising. A vast amount had returned their slip indicating their willingness to carry on further to the interview stage.

Table 6.3 shows the distribution of questionnaires between the different years and incidence of response rates.

The third years' response rate was the lowest out of all three years, the second years' was the highest. Taking the characteristic of 'motivation' to be a precursor of 'readiness' for self-directed learning (Grow, 1991), these results inferred that a similar pattern would emerge with subsequent S.D.L.R.S. scores: third years would be lower than first or second, and second years would demonstrate higher scores than first or third years. This was not necessarily the case as the description of raw scores shows (Table 6. 4).

A score on the S.D.L.R.S. indicates the student's total readiness for self-directed learning at any one time. The maximum score possible on the scale is 290, a minimum is 58, and so an average score is 116 (Guglielmino, 1977).

As can be seen from Table 6.4, all the respondents scored well above the average score of 116. Therefore, even though the first- and third-year student group scored marginally higher and lower scores respectively, differences in 'readiness' between years was negligible. All students were high scorers. This student population appeared to demonstrate an acute degree of 'readiness' for self-direction in their learning.

I could logically conclude that as all 66 students were highly self-directed in their learning, my initial suspicions regarding the third years' learning behaviour were unfounded.

As my knowledge about quantitative data analysis grew, so did my confidence in its instructive capacity, not to mention my own emerging

Table 6.3 Questionnaire distribution and response

	First year	Second year	Third year	N
Total	34	32	39	105
Response	23	23	20	66
%	68	72	51	62

Table 6.4 Description of raw scores within and between years

Year	N	Maximum	Minimum	Mean	Median	Range
First	23	253	180	215	211	73
Second	23	259	142	212	218	117
Third	20	264	170	210	204.5	94

statistical proficiency! I wanted to see what else they could tell me about my student group.

I examined the measure of score dispersion around the mean cores of each year. In other words, I measured the standard deviation (SD) of each group (Table 6.5). The SD would be a more accurate calculation of S.D.L.R.S. scores within and between each student group, and give a more comprehensive picture than a simple descriptive analysis of average scores.

If the SD of a group of scores is large, this implies the range of scores are distributed a long way from the mean. Conversely, if the SD is small most scores occur very close to the average mean, and differences are therefore negligible. A SD of 0 denotes all scores as identical – a SD of 20–25 indicates a wide score distribution (Heyes *et al.*, 1988).

As Table 6.5 shows, all three SDs were comparable, indicating that the scores between each successive year were similarly distributed around the mean. The differences in measures of score dispersion then was minimal.

Thanks to Messers Heyes, Hardy, Humphries and Rookes (1988) I felt equipped to tackle descriptive statistical calculations by hand. Their text was accessible and practical. However, computer packages would have done this for me, had I access to the relative hardware.

A study comprising 66 people is an extremely small population upon which to compare the existence of readiness for self-directed learning between years, but the fact that 100 per cent of S.D.L.R.S. scores happened to be high was in itself astonishing. Could this be true of nursing groups generally? I found it difficult to take on board that I had by chance amassed a group of highly motivated learners. They appeared to be fairly typical of the other students in the college, and so I wanted to examine whether this phenomenon was to be expected with other groups.

My enthusiasm for the subject matter meant that my probing questions had taken me nicely into parametric analysis. This in itself was not a problem, but my population sample was decidedly small for this type of analysis. I needed a non-parametric test that would examine the data generated from a small randomly selected population, that consisted of three variables or subsections – first, second and third year student nurses.

I know this now, and it all sounds so plausible, but at the time I was totally unaware of what I was doing or why. I was having fun – reality was about to hit home!

Table 6.5 Measure of score dispersion within and between groups

Year	Median	Mode	Mean	SD
First	211	–	215	21
Second	218	233	212	26
Third	204	201/197	210	23

Using inferential statistics

There are two types of inferential statistical methods – parametric and non-parametric. As the word indicates, parametric methods estimate parameters of the population, such as the mean. Accuracy of analysis from such methods depends on three main assumptions:

1) scores are drawn from normally distributed populations;
2) two normal distributions have the same variance (the SD squared);
3) the results of the experiment reflect use of interval or ratio data.

Both 1 and 2 depend on a large number of scores randomly drawn from the population.

As my sample was small, distribution was not normal. Distributions would be normal if the mean median and mode had the same values (Heyes *et al.*, 1988). As the median and mode differed in all three groups (Table 6.5) distribution curves would therefore be skewed.

Normally distributed populations would fit the criteria for conducting parametric tests, or one-way analysis of variance (ANOVA) (Siegal and Castellan, 1988). An example of an ANOVA parametric test is the t-test.

Using multiple parametric t-testing to examine differences in *small* groups, with an *unequal distribution of variance* (both these characteristics were explicit in my sample), greatly increases a risk of Type 1 error: the result is said to be significant but later found to be unreliable (Heyes *et al.*, 1988).

Considerations at this stage

I had hit a morass of impenetrable unintelligible information that was insurmountable! My supervisor reassured me that this further analysis was unnecessary, as what I had achieved already was perfectly adequate for the level of course I was on. What course? I had almost lost sight of my degree; I was totally sucked into a fact-finding mission that was rapidly outstripping my intellectual capabilities.

My supervisor's advice was well founded; but I had questions that needed answering. How was it that my students were so highly motivated? Did this occur by chance?

Daunted, but undefeated, I sought out the expert in my own college. Unfortunately my level of statistical expertise meant the gulf between us was all too apparent. Neither of us had the time to spend on this problem – the problem now being not the research itself, but my lack of statistical proficiency and knowledge, and the apparent dearth of available help.

By her own admission, the input I was seeking was above my supervisor's capabilities. I felt deflated and angry, not with anyone personally, but by the lack of academic credibility within my own profession. The educational elocution expounding the importance of research awareness did not appear to exist in reality.

It did not matter that my progress to date was more than adequate for a first degree. I was eating, sleeping and breathing those critical dimensions of learning maturity that I had researched, documented and discovered in others.

As the type of support and concrete assistance I needed at this time did not appear to exist within the profession the answer came from outside; a colleague of my husband's who had a higher degree in mathematics.

I found this person by chance. Not only was his knowledge apparent, but he could understand and relate to the exact nature of my request. I shall be forever indebted to him for his wisdom and patience, as he pedantically explained confusing terms and calculations.

Once the statistical methods were explained, and the correct test identified, it was all relatively straightforward. I just needed someone to show me which combination I should use to unlock the following puzzle: which non-parametric test measures differences between three groups?

By a process of deliberation and elimination, the choice was between one of two – the 'Median' or 'Kruskal–Wallis H' test (Siegal and Castellan, 1988). As the category of my data scores were ordinal rather than nominal or interval, the Kruskal–Wallis H test was the appropriate analysis to use (Siegal and Castellan, 1988; Polgar and Thomas, 1991).

The Kruskal–Wallis H test

This test is the most powerful non-parametric test for examining three or more (k) independent samples in a 'between-subject' design (Siegal and Castellan, 1988).

It has a power efficiency of 95.5 per cent of the ANOVA, or F test, to detect existing differences *between* groups (Siegal and Castellan, 1988). In other words, accuracy of this test was comparable to parametric tests.

The technique tests a *null* hypothesis, that is there will be *no* differences between variables: *the sum of the ranks for each group are approximately equal* so *there is no difference in S.D.L.R.S. scores between years.*

As there were more than five subjects per sample, a chi-square table was used to determine the levels of significance.

If a null hypothesis, indicated as H(o), is *greater* than or *equal* to the table value of chi-square distribution, the groups are considered statistically different, and so the null hypothesis can be rejected (Heyes *et al.*, 1988; Siegal and Castellan, 1988): there is a statistical difference in S.D.L.R. scores between years.

The degrees of freedom (df) relate to the number of scores that are theoretically free to vary given the other existing scores and their sum total

Table 6.6 Kruskal–Wallis ANOVA for between-subject analysis

Year	df	H(o)	Chi-squared	P
First/third	17	18.97	27.59	0.05
First/second	21	21.99	32.67	0.05
Second/third	17	18.96	27.59	0.05
Second/third	17	18.97	27.59	0.05*

*adjusted for ties

(Heyes *et al.*, 1988). Degrees of freedom are calculated at the 5 per cent significant level (*P*).

Results

The Kruskal–Wallis non-parametric method of analysis tested a combination of between-subject independent observations, against a table value of chi-square at $P = 0.05$, with 17 df (Table 6.6). The return value of chi-square against H(o) was greater in all four examples (comparing second and third year twice, once adjusted for ties). Therefore, the null hypothesis is accepted: *there is no statistical difference* in readiness for self-directed learning between first, second and third year students; a relationship between *readiness for self-directed learning and student seniority in this sample group does not exist.*

Although these results are 95.5 per cent significant, its significance is relative to this study, and as such can not be generalized. But, my results had not occurred by chance. All the students in my sample exhibited self-directed learning behaviours. If this randomly selected student group were high scorers, it was probable that the findings would be similar in replicated studies.

As Clarke and Dickenson (1976), Oddi (1986) and Emblen and Gray (1990) attest, nurses are self-directed learners, therefore their sense of readiness for this type of learning is already established.

Considering that all scores within the sample group were above average (116), it is not surprising that a Kruskal–Wallis ANOVA concluded that a null hypothesis can not be rejected: *there was no statistical difference in readiness for self-directed learning between any of the three years.* A relationship between readiness for self-directed learning and student seniority did not exist. The non-parametric analysis corroborated findings from descriptive review.

My supervisor was correct in her advice that the initial analysis was quite sufficient. However, results from both types of analysis validated findings, and so gave weight to the scientific merit of my study. Therefore I still feel justified in what I set out to do, and conquered (with a little help – granted).

The experience has not lessened my enthusiasm for using this type of approach in the future. I gained more than I lost. It exposed a whole new world of informatics that I knew existed but was afraid to acknowledge. I have since gained an understanding of the scope of its potential, as information technology is increasingly becoming a necessary facet of professional life.

Considerations at this stage

- Be sure exactly how statistics are to address the purpose of the study. It could be too late to try and think about this once the data is collected.
- Background information on basic statistics is essential for an informed decision as to the application of types of analysis. This very much relates to the research purpose.
- Investigating the geographical location of essential resources includes:
  a) a usable statistics book with a comprehensive glossary;
  b) expert advice and/or knowledge that can be easily accessed such as computer software that is appropriate to the level and type of analysis required.

Limitations and recommendations

Limitations

Two limiting factors pertinent to the study's methodology were content validity – inconsistencies within the population, and construct validity – inappropriate choice of method and design (Heyes *et al.*, 1988).

Content validity

Analysis of the distribution of responses between the three student groups demonstrated that the third years' lowest response rate was disproportionate to their largest sample size.

Throughout the study, I was advised by work colleagues that this particular year were 'a bad lot', and therefore not a good choice to sample. Finding another third year group would have been impossible within the college at such short notice. Fortunately, personal experience with the year meant I was not unduly concerned as I was sure our relationship would stand me in good stead – it did.

However, subsequent interviews with members of the group revealed blatant hostility directed toward the college. As I was seen to represent the establishment, this hostility was initially targeted at myself; hence the small response rate.

Cohen and Manion (1983) purport that attitudes and expectations teachers hold towards people they teach considerably affect student responses. A teacher's attitude towards their students may initiate a self-fulfilling prophecy. Whereas 'teaching' may be a 'vastly over-rated function' (Rogers, 1969, 1972, cited in Jones, 1981, p. 60), teachers are not.

It is interesting, in the light of Cohen and Manion's (1983) comments, that the third years' behaviour was as other teachers had expected – uncooperative, de-motivated and hostile.

The students' overwhelming complaint was that, as a group, they were unable to relate to the majority of staff. This resulted in their feelings of isolation from the college culture. This antagonism was reflected in negative learning behaviours and interfered with factor analysis regarding readiness for self-direction in learning. As such the population's 'internal consistency' was suspect.

Recommendation 1

The change from dependence to independence is not sequential, as there is no one good way to manage everyone. But, everyone can be managed in such a way that increases an ability to be self-directed. The outcome of this behaviour is strongly influenced by the teacher's attitude inherent in their 'style' of teaching (Fischer and Fischer, 1979).

The overwhelming factor qualitative analysis revealed was the effect this teaching style had in determining readiness for self-directed learning. The degree of openness and trust in an educational relationship has a direct effect on the learners' perception of themselves, their attitude to learning and the quality of care patients receive.

Asymmetrical power relations between teachers and students are likely to be mirrored through nurse–patient interactions. This does not underpin a humanistic paradigm subsumed within nursing's philosophy.

It is therefore unfair to expect any student automatically to adopt adult learning behaviours and attitudes. Educational maturity is a phenomenon that needs to be nurtured; it is a learning strategy that is distinctly situational, and so should be encouraged on an individual basis.

Good teaching then matches the learner's stage of self-direction and helps the learner advance toward greater independence in learning.

Construct validity

Assessing a person's readiness for self-directed learning through quasi-experimental approaches was inappropriate. If people are willing to set time aside, read, fill in the questionnaire and post it back on time, then surely these people are already demonstrating motivation and cooperation. Perhaps this is the reason why all scores within the sample group were well above average – those people keen to complete the questionnaire were highly likely to be motivated learners. If not, would they be bothered to complete the questionnaire in the first place? My choice of design and method would automatically skew the results of the data. Not much wonder then the results were so startling!

What I needed was a cross–sample of the students; but this would have been difficult to obtain. The alternative would have been to stand over unwilling participants to ensure they complied with my wishes. Although this would enhance the quality of population sample, this would do very little to enhance the study's reliability of data or, for that matter, ethical motives!

Vollmer (1986) explored the relationship between expectancy and academic achievement:

> A fundamental assumption in all theories of achievement motivation is thus, that expectancy is an adequate determinant of motivational activation which, in turn, influences quality of performance. (p. 65)

Therefore, a student's perceived level of learning ability has consequences for their level of motivation, which in turn affects performance. In other words, the students' expectation of failure influenced their decision to participate in the study – those that did participate, expected to score well, and they were not disappointed. Therefore all my students would inevitably be ready to take on board self-directed learning experiences. I am left wondering if a very different picture would have emerged from students who did not return their questionnaires.

This method was totally inappropriate for what I wanted to find out. My initial analysis had not actually revealed anything. The choice of method had completely invalidated my initial results!

Recommendation 2

In view of the study's major methodological limitations, examining readiness for self-directed learning in future should be through qualitative rather than quantitative studies. A phenomenological approach would minimize the chance of expectancy, motivation and performance (Vollmer, 1986) to contaminate results.

Conclusion

Although the choice of method, and idiosyncracies within the third year group had profound implications for the quality of my study overall, by this stage I was unassailable. The learning curve I had surmounted was phenomenal. I was so proud of what I had managed to achieve that the whole experience was reward enough. As an inexperienced teacher the study had helped me understand myself, the students I taught and the various learning processes involved. In short it was an empowering experience.

On completing the study I began to perceive the enormity of my professional responsibilities. My teaching style influenced the quality of relationship with my students, which in turn directly affected their degree of readiness for self-directed learning.

A teaching style that generated open, collaborative atmospheres in any learning situation would cultivate critical thinking abilities. As a nurse educator, I needed to enhance teaching strategies that would foster students' critical reflective skills, not self-direction. I had been barking up the wrong tree.

Critical reflection is a skill that precedes readiness for self-directed learning. A nurse who exhibits self-directed learning behaviours is ready to be open and receptive to new and exciting developments in nursing. Readiness assures the presence of practical capabilities in order to participate in the creation of evolving forms of nursing care, relevant to the diversified contextual situations in which students find themselves.

Critically reflective practitioners can articulate clear and informed rationale as to why they do what they do, justify their decisions and make sound clinical judgements. This professional integrity is vital in lieu of political initiatives that emphasize cost above quality. Unless we can prove our academic solidarity by grasping educational opportunities inherent in P.R.E.P., nurses could find themselves priced out of a job!

Although it is now five years since I completed my research, this single piece of work epitomized the agony and the ecstasy of actually doing a degree level course. To name but a few: late nights, writer's cramp, midnight telephone calls, photocopying bills, developing and testing lifelong relationships, insight, transformation and empowerment.

Despite the problems I encountered from choosing to complete an empirical study, I do not regret my decision. I have never considered myself particularly academic and so the surge of surprise and pride in obtaining the highest classification possible was immense. Granted, the work I produced was above that required for my level of degree, but this was not what I had intended at the outset.

As the study progressed, I began to experience a personal education that was so tangible at times it almost hurt. The pain never exceeded the pleasure I received from the whole experience, and this was entirely due to formal and informal support networks. This was the most important lesson of all: do not underestimate the importance of supervision or friends.

The relationship I had with my supervisor meant our meetings were high impact encounters, that required pre-planning and a good deal of subsequent effort on my part. They were also fun. It also requires effort, planning and a sense of humour on the supervisor's part, but such was the level of my stress, I was completely oblivious to her skills. Supervision is not an innate quality, and I have since learned to perfect this process by remembering and valuing her expertise.

The second important lesson was to be organized, not only with data but, more importantly, with time. This meant starting early. I was amazed as to how long it actually took before I had a focus for my research: at least four months – one to choose a topic area, and three to read around the subject. This was before I had my title and could start systematically combing the literature. Giving myself adequate time also meant that when things got hot under the collar, I was not pressurized by deadlines. Time on my side meant I had space to work through unforeseen problems, the main one being getting stuck in a mire of inferential statistics.

A final lesson, which I did not benefit from at the time, was keeping it all in perspective. This is something I have subsequently managed to instil in my own research students. Personal experience of supervision has shown that if all is well the student is normally in a continual state of low-level panic. This keeps them moving forward, and ensures targets and goals are achieved. However, the intensity involved in studying for this type of assessment can lead to burn-out. As with my own study, if the learning experience becomes personal then students are too much a part of the process to recognize its all-consuming nature. For this reason, keeping the experience in perspective is the supervisor's responsibility rather than the student's. This is easily articulated, but is by far the most difficult and challenging aspect to implement.

Some final considerations at this stage

I believe that nursing research has two purposes: to gain the kind of knowledge that will help practitioners improve their practice, and to gain a deeper understanding of the nature of nursing. Different research methods are simply different ways of seeing and thinking, sometimes about the same thing. Each one potentiates the other in order to give a more complete picture of the phenomena being studied. Given that each is used appropriately, one is neither better nor worse than the other. To suggest otherwise defends and preserves a hierarchy of knowledge.

Nursing is establishing its scientific foundations in order to guide the artistry of practice. Utilizing established deductive theories in various nursing models is complemented by inductive processes nurses are beginning to use to reveal knowledge buried in practice. The taken for granted aspects of nurses' daily work contains a wealth of information about the uniqueness of individuals and the totality of human beings. This knowledge is brought to light by the highly personal activity of reflection. Combining these different approaches to knowledge through education and research blends the science and art of nursing in such a way that the uniqueness of our practice is clearly expressed (Carper, 1978; Visintainer, 1986; Peplau, 1988).

Reflective processes have great potential for investigating aspects of our work which can not be easily explained or articulated. Recognition of this fact is now becoming more established both within and outside the profession (MacPhearson, 1983; Thompson, 1987; Rosser, 1988; Wilkinson, 1988; Campbell and Bunting, 1991; Taylor, 1993). Among positivist, rational scientists however, its contribution to a wider sphere of knowledge is not recognized or encouraged on the basis of its degree of subjectivity (Acker *et al.*, 1983; Stacey, 1988).

While this polemic will run for a while yet, I see the use of reflective methods becoming more prevalent in nursing research, and at last ending the qualitative/quantitative debate. For this to occur practitioners and teachers must make a conscious effort to refine their reflective skills, as well as demonstate that this process of enlightenment is underpinned with scientific intelligence. In this way we can be sure that nursing science is nourished by the artistry of our craft.

My own experience attests to the fact that there is a dearth of 'scientific' expertise within the profession. The growing number of nursing students undertaking degree courses will inevitably develop all aspects of nursing knowledge through research, including knowledge gleaned through traditional science. It is my belief that researcher supervision must come from within the profession for the science of the nurse's craft to remain practice focused. A 'practical science' develops techniques to solve practical problems while an 'applied science' uses existing theories to solve practical problems (Johnson, 1991).

Nursing is a practice based profession. The science that guides and supports our craft should be both applied and practised. In this way, we can be sure that nursing theory is generated from inductive as well as deductive knowledge. If, however, students are constantly having to seek supervision from people other than nurses, how can we truely develop a science that is essentially about nursing? At best, nursing science would be applied to, rather than generated from practice. Totally relying on knowledge external to the discipline in order to understand and explain the world around us, specifically one focused on nursing, does little to enhance professional, academic or practical kudos. I would argue that unless we develop our scientific as well as our artistic expertise our accolade for nursing having a unique knowledge base will be no more than rhetoric.

References

Acker J, Barry J and Esseveld J (1983) Objectivity and truth: problems in doing feminist research. *Womens Studies International Forum* 6 (4), 423–35.

Bell J (1987) *Doing Your Research Project – A Guide for the First Time Researchers in Education and Social Science*. Open University Press, Milton Keynes.

Benton D C and Cormack D F S (1991) Reviewing and evaluating the literature. In Cormack D F S (Ed.) *The Research Process in Nursing*. Blackwell Scientific Publications, Oxford.

Box B J (1983) Self-directed learning readiness of students and graduates of an associated degree nursing programme. *Dissertation Abstracts International* 44, 697–a.

Brockett R G (1985) The relationship between self-directed learning and life satisfaction among older adults. *Adult Education Quaterly* 35 (4), 210–19.

Brookfield S (1988) *Training Educators of Adults*.

Bruner J S (1966) *Towards a Theory of Instruction*. Belknapp, Cambridge, MA.

Burnard P (1989) Experiential learning and andragogy – negotiated learning in nurse education. *Nurse Education Today* 9 (5), 300–6.

Burnard P (1990) The student experience: adult learning and mentorship revisited. *Nurse Education Today* 10 (5), 349–54.

Burns N and Grove S K (1987) *The Practice of Nursing Research: Conduct Critique and Utilisation*. W B Saunders, Philadelphia.

Carper B (1978) Fundamental patterns of knowing in nursing. *Advances in Nursing Science*, 1 (1), 13–23.

Campbell J C and Bunting S (1991) Voices and paradigms: perspectives on critical and feminist theory in nursing. *Advances in Nursing Science* 13 (3), 1–15.

Chinn P L and Kramer M K (1991) *Theory and Nursing. A Systematic Approach*, 3rd edn. Mosby Year Books, St Louis.

Clarke K M and Dickenson G (1976) Self directed and other directed continuing education: A study of nurses participation. *Journal of Continuing Education in Nursing* 7 (4), 16–24.

Cohen L and Manion L (1983) *A Guide to Teaching Practice*, 2nd edn. Methuen, London.

Cohen L and Manion L (1989) *Research Methods in Education*, 3rd edn. Routledge, London.

Conti G J (1985) The relationship between teaching style and adult student learning. *Adult Education Quarterly* 35 (4), 220–8.

Cooper S S (1978) Self-directed learning. *Journal of Continuing Education in Nursing* 9 (1), 5–6.

Cormack D F S (1991) *The Research Process in Nursing*. Blackwell Scientific Publications, Oxford.

Crook J (1985) A validation study of a self-directed learning readiness scale. *Journal of Nursing Education* 24 (7), September 274–9.

Donnan P T (1991) Quantitative analysis: (Inferential) In Cormack D F S (Ed.) *The Research Process in Nursing*. Blackwell Scientific, Oxford, Chapter 28.

Emblen J D and Gray G T (1990) Comparsion of nurses self-directed learning activities. *Journal of Continuing Education in Nursing* 21 (2), 56–61.

Fischer B B and Fischer L (1979) Styles in teaching and learning. *Educational Leadership* 36 (4), 245–54.

Goodwin L D and Goodwin W L (1984) Qualitative versus quantitative Goodwin research. An attempt to clarify the issues. *Educational Research* 33 (6), 378–80.

Goulbourne A (1992) Is there a relationship between the readiness for self direction in learning and increasing student seniority? Unpublished Dissertation, Stienbeck Collection, R.C.N.

Grow G (1991) Teaching learners to be self directed. *Adult Education Quarterly* 41 (3), 125–46.

Guglielmino L M (1977) Development of the self-directed learning readiness scale. University Microfilms International Dissertation Services.

Hamilton L and Gregor F M (1986) Self-directed learning in a critical care nursing programme. *Journal of Continuing Education in Nursing* 17 (3), May 94–9.

Heyes S, Hardy M, Humphreys P and Rookes P (1988) *Starting Statistics in Psychology and Education – A Student Handbook*. Weidenfeld & Nicolson, London.

Heath J (1979) A new kind of nurse – tomorrow's approach to learning. *Nursing Mirror* 149 (6), 9 August 22–3.

Hollingworth S (1980) Teaching the nursing process. In Richardson M (Ed.) Innovating andragogy in a basic nursing course: an evaluation of the self-directed independent study contract with basic nursing students. *Nurse Education Today* 8 (6), 315–24.

Iwasiw C L (1987) The role of the teacher in self-directed learning. *Nurse Education Today* 7 October, 222–7.

Johnson J L (1991) Nursing science: basic applied or practical? Implications for the art of nursing. *Advances in Nursing Science* 14 (1), 7–16.

Jones W (1981) Self-directed learning and student selected goals in nurse education. *Journal of Advanced Nursing* 6, 59–69.

Katherein M A (1982) A study of self-directed continued professional learning members of Illinois Nurses Association: Content and process. Doctoral Dissertation. *Dissertation Abstracts International* 42, 1902–a.

Knowles M S (1973) *The Modern Practice of Adult Education*. Association Press, New York, Chapters 1 and 3.

Knowles M S (1978) *The Adult Learner: A Neglected Species*, 2nd edn. Gulf Publishing, Houston, TX.

Kuschinkas V (1979) Whose cognitive style makes the difference? *Educational Leadership* 36, 269–71.

Lancaster A (1975) An introduction to the research process (2). Guidelines to research in nursing. Occasional Papers. *Nursing Times* 22 May, 45–8.

Long H B and Agyekum S (1984) Guglielmino's self-directed learning readiness scale: a validation study. *Higher Education* 12, 77–87.

Marriner A (1980) Research design: Survey/descriptive. In Krampitz S D and Pavlovich I (Eds) *Readings for Nursing Research*. Mosby, St Louis, Chapter 4.

Macphearson K L (1983) Feminist methods: a new paradigm for nursing research. *Advances in Nursing Science* January, 17–25.

Oddi L F (1986) Development and validation of an instrument to identify self-directed continuing learners. *Adult Education Quarterly* 36 (2), 97–107.

O'Kell S P (1988) A study of the relationship between learning style, readiness for self-directed learning and teaching preference of learner nurses in one health district. *Nurse Education Today* 8, 197–204.

Peplau H E (1988) The art and science of nursing. Similarities, differences and relations. *Nursing Science Quarterly* 1 (1), 8–15.

Polgar S and Thomas S A (1991) *Introduction to Research in Health Sciences*, 2nd edn. Churchill Livingstone, Edinburgh.

Richardson M (1988) Innovating andragogy in a basic nursing course: an evaluation of the self-directed independent study contract with basic nursing students. *Nurse Education Today* 8, 315–24.

Rosser V (1988) Good science, can it ever be gender free? *Women's Studies International Forum* 11 (1), 13–19.

Stacey J (1988) Can there be a feminist ethnography? *Women's Studies International Forum* 6 (4), 423–35.

Siegal S and Castellan N J (1988) *Non Parametric Statistics for the Behavioural Sciences*, 2nd edn. Churchill Livingstone, Edinburgh.

Sweeney J F (1986) Nurse education: learner centred or teacher centred. *Nurse Education Today* 6 (6), 257–62.

Savoie M L (1980) Continuing education for nurses: predictors of success in courses requiring a degree of learning self-direction. *Dissertation Abstracts International* 40, 6114–a.

Skaggs B J (1981) The relationship between involvement of professional nurses in self-directed learning, loci of control and readiness for self-directed measures. *Dissertation Abstracts International* 42, 1906–a.

Taylor J S (1993) Resolving epistemological pluralism: a personal account of the research process. *Journal of Advanced Nursing* 18, 1073–6.

Thompson J Z (1987) Critical scholarship: the critique of domination in nursing. *Advances in Nursing Science* January 17–25.

Torrance E P and Mourad S (1978) Some creativity and style of learning and thinking correlates of Guglielmino's self-directed learning readiness scale. *Psychological Reports* 43, 1167–71.

Visintainer M V (1986) The nature of knowledge and theory in nursing. *Image – Journal of Nursing Scholarship* 18 (2), 32–8.

Vollmer F (1986) The relationship between expectancy and academic achievement – how can it be explained? *British Journal of Educational Psychology* 56, 64–74.

Wilkinson S (1988) The role of reflexivity in feminist psychology. *Women's Studies International Forum* 11 (5), 493–502.

Wiley K (1983) Effects of a self-directed learning project and preference for structure on self-directed learning readiness. *Nursing Research* 32 (3), 181–5.

7

The lived experience of phenomenology

Susan Mullaney

Phenomenology is at the extreme opposite end of a continuum of research approaches from quantitative methods:

- *strong belief systems and values on research of nursing emerge in this chapter as the account of this project develops;*
- *the chapter, like Chapter 2, suggests stages both to the research approach but also vital steps to the analysis of data. These are explored in the philosophical context of phenomenology;*
- *the use of written accounts is an approach which lends itself to use in other research contexts;*
- *the references contain essential classics in this approach;*
- *finally, this chapter must be read, and compared with, the next chapter.*

Introduction

Merleau-Ponty (1962) remarked that we can only really understand phenomenology by doing it. Within this chapter I aim to provide a vicarious means of gaining the experience of 'doing' phenomenological research. The chapter commences by exploring the philosophical origin of phenomenology and progresses to an unfolding of the essence of the phenomenological research approach. Within this, Colaizzi's (1978) framework is used to guide data gathering and analysis. Description of the method is limited where a suitable text would suffice. The congruence of the assumptions of phenomenology with those of nursing is examined.

The reader is invited to scrutinize my own research, entitled 'The Post-Registration Students' Perception of High Quality Education in the Classroom'. This is introduced to show one way of 'doing it' and alternatives are offered. Above all, the chapter is intended to explore practical issues and possibly offer some tips for survival when considering this approach for your own research; and as such this is a 'how to'. Throughout the research process reflection was facilitated by a research diary using Boud *et al.*'s (1985) model, shown in Figure 7.1. This proved invaluable, and is woven throughout the chapter.

When writing this chapter, I encountered some of the difficulties identified by Webb (1992), when attempting to verbalize my own lived experience while writing something academically credible. As a result I have chosen to use the first person throughout.

Phenomenology in context

Qualitative methodology focuses on the process of understanding human experience rather than seeking to control or predict it (Burnard and Morrison, 1990). Leininger (1985) describes qualitative research as documenting and interpreting as fully as possible the totality of whatever is being studied, in particular contexts, from the people's viewpoint, or frame of reference. This includes the identification, study and analysis of subjective and objective data in order to understand people's worlds. Qualitative research is carried out within broad theoretical notions about the phenomena under study, using inductive reasoning to derive knowledge from the data generated or collected.

Phenomenology is a philosophy, a research approach and a methodology (Cohen, 1987). It attempts to study the human experience as it is lived (Merleau-Ponty, 1964), accepting that experience as it exists in the consciousness of an individual, complete with meanings and realities (Field and Morse, 1985). It is a viable and valuable qualitative research methodology (Omery, 1983).

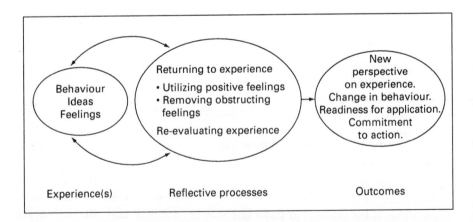

Figure 7.1   A model of reflection (Boud *et al.*, 1985)

Phenomenological inquiry strives to answer the question of 'what is it like?', by insightful description of the way human beings experience the world. The goal is to describe, as truthfully as possible, the phenomenon being studied and not the generation of models or theories (Field and Morse, 1985). Van Manen (1984) suggests that phenomenology aims to come to a deeper understanding of the nature or meaning of our everyday experience, and when describing phenomenology chooses the term 'thoughtfulness'. This thoughtfulness is described as a caring attunement to what it means to live a life. Phenomenological research is a search for what it means to be human, a search for the fullness of living. It is not enough, however, just to recall all those experiences.

Pallikkathayil and Morgan (1991) describe phenomenology as an obsessive search for true understanding of phenomena from the experiencing person's perspective. Success is dependent on an openness to the totality of the phenomenon being studied and a willingness to give credence to the participant's disclosure of the experience (Pallikkathayil and Morgan, 1991). The researcher must be insightful, reflective and intuitive, and phenomenology is therefore not open for all to use. Phenomenology is a way of thinking and a way of being, it is this researcher's usual belief system and way of life. The experiences of phenomenology must be recalled in such a way that the essential aspects, the meaning structure of these experiences as lived through, are brought back. The story is told in such a way that we recognize this description as a human experience. It is one possible interpretation of that experience. The aim is to construct a possible interpretation of the nature of that certain experience, which is a possible interpretation for anyone reading it.

Origins

Phenomenology has developed as a result of positivistic scientific methods, with their emphasis on objectivity, verifiability and repeatability, failing adequately to explain the phenomena of the human being or to take into account their experience (Omery, 1983; Salsberry, 1989). This approach also fails to take into account the 'context dependent' nature of human beings, their actions and experiences (Munhall and Oiler, 1986).

The subjective experience, which was eliminated from the objective scientific experiment, was beginning to be perceived as more basic and real in the understanding of human knowledge and behaviour, than experimental data (Omery, 1983). Husserl, a German mathematician, is said to have established phenomenology and, subsequently, the value of phenomenology as a research method for understanding and explaining human experience began to be recognized (Omery, 1983).

Phenomenology as a research method has grown out of the philosophical movement. The philosophy is still being clarified, and as a result many interpretations of phenomenological method can be found in the literature (Van Kaam, 1959, 1966; Giorgi, 1970; Colaizzi, 1978; van Manen, 1984; Parse *et al.*, 1986); however, they share the common goal of describing the essential structure of the phenomenon, differing in the process used to arrive at that essential structure. Spiegelberg (1960), the historian of phenomenological philosophy, identified six steps believed to be common to all interpretations of the philosophical method (Figure 7.2). Those who have described and implemented the research method have been influenced by these steps rather than applying them (Omery, 1983). Van Manen (1984) offers four elements of methodological activity (Figure 7.3) which facilitate this data driven research.

The research method, underpinned by the philosophical assumptions of phenomenology, accepts experience as it exists in the consciousness of an individual complete with subjective meanings and realities (Field and Morse, 1985). Phenomenology endeavours, through an inductive, descriptive method, to study the human experience as it is lived (Oiler, 1982). Participants' descriptions, or stories of their experiences, are analysed to uncover meaning and promote an understanding of human beings.

Phenomenology for nursing

Phenomenology, with its focus on human phenomena, is a method consistent with the values and beliefs of a humanistic discipline such as nursing

1. Descriptive phenomenology: direct investigation, analysis, and description of the phenomena under study, as free as possible from preconceived expectations and presuppositions.

2. Phenomenology of the essences: perception and probing of the phenomena for typical structures or 'essentials' and for the relationship of the structures.

3. Phenomenology of appearances: giving attention to or watching for the ways phenomena appear in different perspectives or modes of clarity, that is, determining the distinct from the hazy surrounding it.

4. Constituitive phenomenology: exploring the constitution or the way in which the phenomenon establishes itself or takes shape in consciousness.

5. Reductive phenomenology: suspending belief in the reality or validity of the phenomena: a process that has been implicit since the inception of the method now becomes explicit through the use of the technique of 'bracketing', which can be defined as 'detaching the phenomena of our everyday experience from the context of our naive or natural living, while preserving the content as fully as possible.

6. Hermeneutic phenomenology: interpreting the concealed meanings in the phenomena that are not immediately revealed to direct investigation, analysis and description.

Figure 7.2 Steps of phenomenological philosophy (after Spiegelberg, 1960)

1. Turning to a phenomenon which seriously interests us and commits us to the world.

2. Investigating experience as we live it rather than as we conceptualize it.

3. Reflecting on the essential themes which characterize the phenomenon.

4. Describing the phenomenon through the art of writing and re-writing.

Figure 7.3 Four methodological activities (after van Manen, 1984)

(Benner, 1985; Lynch-Sauer, 1985; Munhall and Oiler, 1986). Nursing has become increasingly committed to the appropriateness of qualitative methodologies for the study of nursing phenomena (Parse, 1981; Haase, 1987; Watson, 1988; Bennett, 1991; Beck, 1992, Appleton, 1993). As nursing practice involves the diagnosis, caring for, and treatment of human responses to actual and potential health problems, and since humans respond as whole persons, knowledge of the lived experiences of health are legitimate topics of nursing research (Swanson-Kauffman and Schonwald, 1988). The approach is said to be suited to the study of the more elusive concepts that characterize concerns in nursing practice (Munhall and Oiler, 1986). Providing holistic care has become a concern in the recent past and is presented as a selling point in the marketing of health care.

Often the methodology of health-related research originated with the physical sciences. Problems of health and illness are approached in a reductionist way that fragments people, labelling them into parts that are biological, sociological, or psychological components of human beings. If we are serious about humanizing health care and making holistic care available to patients and clients, and their families, then we need to expand our research methods to fit this holistic task (Drew, 1989).

Phenomenological research has begun to ask what it means to be a patient. It provides the opportunity to consider what human experience means and, within this context, the researcher's subjective experience can also be important (Drew, 1989). One of the strengths of phenomenology is that it takes into account the relationship between the researcher and the phenomenon (Drew, 1989). Nursing practice offers a rich source of human experience suitable for investigation using the phenomenological method and can include the nurse's lived experience as well as that of the client or patient. Nurses who want to increase their understanding of a given lived experience can use phenomenological method to gain that understanding within their everyday practice.

Research in context

My own research study, introduced in this chapter, was a course requirement for an Honours degree. At that time, I was employed as course lecturer to the English National Board (ENB) Course 998, Teaching and Assessing in Clinical Practice. I was not enthralled with the prospect of undertaking research, and had an alternative been available to me, I would have taken it. It was not until I studied a compulsory research methods module that my own interest in phenomenology began to spark. The reason for this lack of enthusiasm, I believed, lay with the closed language of research, the overwhelming fear of statistics, coupled with a failure to see their relevance, and a lack of ability to be critical. I now believe that I was ignorant of the process, an admission which came long after the advent of research based practice. I therefore approached the project as a research novice.

My research took place at a time of rapid change in nurse education both nationally and locally. Historically, following the circulation of the outline curriculum document for Course 998 (National Boards of England and Wales, 1985), many Schools of Nursing recognized the significance of this course. The curriculum was devised in response to the growing wealth of research into the clinical learning environment, which suggested that qualified nurses were ill-prepared for their roles as teachers, supervisors and assessors of learners in clinical environments.

The aim of the course is to help staff involved in teaching, supervising and assessing students to develop further appreciation and understanding of the process of learning; to gain enhanced knowledge and improved skills in the fundamental aspects of teaching and assessing, and to create a supportive learning environment in the clinical areas (National Boards for England and Wales, 1985). The underlying philosophy for the course included the concepts of teaching and learning as a shared process, with the ultimate responsibility resting with the course students to initiate and sustain their own professional development. The students were regarded as adult learners. The major responsibility of the teacher, therefore, was to create a supportive learning environment.

As course lecturer to ENB Course 998, Teaching and Assessing in Clinical Practice, I believed that the course significantly influenced and publicized the reputation of the college for high quality education. These students have gained further appreciation and understanding of the process of learning, and how to create supportive learning environments, and therefore are more able than other qualified nurses to be critical of the quality of education provision. These were the students who, in their roles as nurses and managers, would be individually purchasing continuing education for themselves and contracting to purchase continuing education in the future.

For these reasons, I believed it was important that a supportive learning environment, where high quality education in the classroom could take place, was ensured, but first I had to understand what the students' experience was.

Stages of the process

The stages that I progressed through from identifying the focus of the study to the presentation of the findings, now follow as an illustration of the process. It is important to use a time-plan for the staging of this process (Field and Morse, 1985). This ensures sufficient time will be allotted to the not insignificant task of reflecting on themes, theme clusters and theme categories as they emerge, and to put aside the study prior to writing and rewriting.

The costs of undertaking traditional research studies are not involved with phenomenology, however there are hidden costs, such as a good tape-recorder, a secretary to transcribe the recordings and much paper. In one study the transcribed interviews yielded 686 double-spaced pages, of 20 to 52 pages per interview (Pallikkathayil and Morgan, 1991).

Features of the New Paradigm Research (Reason and Rowan, 1981), in which co-operative enquiry is advocated as an approach, researching 'with' participants rather than 'on' them, is congruent with the assumptions of phenomenology and is worthy of consideration at this point.

Research question

The starting point of phenomenological research is in the identification of something that is deeply interesting, and the verification of this interest as a true phenomenon, that is, an experience that human beings live through. The nature and number of human experiences are infinite. At the beginning of my study, I had some notions of the general direction along which it might evolve and develop, rather than a specific research question. I hoped that it would allow me to explore the experience of high quality classroom education for post-registration students.

The methodology used evolved as the study progressed. This exploratory approach, with plans, ideas and informal structure rather than fixed formal structure and boundaries, is typical of qualitative research (Field and Morse, 1985). I hoped, as the research progressed, that the methodology would be driven by the data, and that I would be open to new ideas and be flexible within the chosen approach (Patton, 1980). This would allow me to develop from the experience of learning new theories and putting theories into practice. I wanted to learn with and through the research.

I approached the Research Approval Panel of my then employing College for permission to carry out the study by submitting a proposal, following their guidelines and outlining my intentions. The Panel required that I made the purpose of the study and the methodology more explicit, with specific research procedure.

Patton (1980) informs the novice researcher wishing to use the phenomenological method that, for the research to be truly phenomenological in nature, one must not develop a set of steps, but must proceed as the direction of the experience indicates, without the restrictions such a structure would impose. The novice researcher should explore the meaning of that experience as it unfolds for the participant. This I had to compromise to progress the study. This validated James' (1992) comments in 'A Postscript to Nursing' where she states that her proposal was deliberately left flexible so that there was room to manoeuvre, but this was interpreted as not knowing what she was doing. Following clarification concerning the methodology, support for the study was given. The flexibility of the process and the reluctance on the part of the phenomenological researcher to specify an end-product, can be interpreted as a poor knowledge base by those more used to quantitative studies.

An important reminder at this point is to be aware of the original question throughout the work, and to be constantly orientated to the chosen lived experience that makes you ask what is it like in the first place. Gadamer (1975) stated that the essence of the question is the opening up, and keeping open, of possibilities. We can only do this if we are open to the question which concerns us ourselves. We need to 'live' the question and become that question. The clearer and less ambiguous the question the less ambiguous the interpretation of the research findings (van Manen, 1984).

The phenomenological researcher must entice the reader into the question, so that the reader cannot help but wonder about it. It can be said that phenomenological questioning itself teaches the reader to wonder and to question deeply.

Bracketing

One of the problems of phenomenological enquiry is not that we know too little about a subject that interests us deeply, it is that we know too much. Or more accurately that our common sense, assumptions and existing knowledge predispose us to interpret the nature of the phenomenon before we have come to grips with the question. It is difficult to ignore or to forget what we already know, and it is an impossible ideal to expect a researcher to do so. It is my knowledge, beliefs, biases and assumptions that make me the individual that I now am with an interest in high quality classroom education and a growing persuasion to the delights of phenomenology. It is better, therefore, to make these assumptions, beliefs, understandings, biases and theories explicit and to expose them.

The importance in a phenomenological study of suspending our own beliefs and assumptions about the phenomena undergoing exploration is recognized, and referred to as bracketing (van Manen, 1984). To ensure that the phenomenon is being investigated as it is truly experienced, a necessary criterion is that the researcher must approach the phenomenon to be explored with no preconceived expectations (Omery, 1983). The researcher is not seeking to validate a predetermined theoretical framework or collect data to fit existing literature.

There are many ways to attempt to achieve bracketing. My assumptions, beliefs and biases were discovered as the research took place. The best means of bracketing, I believed, was to undertake a written account in the same way as the participants.

Bracketing may also be realized by the researcher undertaking to complete any of the data gathering exercises proposed for their own participants, for example, being interviewed or keeping a diary. Bracketing, in common with intuiting, appears to enhance the trustworthiness of the method and contributes to its rigour.

Ethical considerations

I followed a number of overall principles while undertaking this study, as I believe ethical principles are more than successful approval from an Ethics Committee. These are included as I believe they contribute to the rigour of the methodology:

- The well-being of the participants took precedence over the aims and processes of the study.
- All participants were made aware of their right to anonymity, confidentiality and to withdraw at any time.
- Anonymity for each participant returning a completed a written account was offered, leaving it optional whether participants identified themselves or not.
- Confidentiality of authorship of statements by participants was assured throughout. All participants were reassured that information in the report could not identify them personally.
- Security of the written accounts was guaranteed. These were kept in a locked file when not in use. The secretary used to transcribe the interviews was informed that these transcripts and the information contained within were confidential. The secretary did not have access to the codes linking names to numbers, nor did she know any of the interviewees and therefore would not recognize voices from the cassette tapes. For the interviews, which were audiotape recorded, I used written consent, adapted from Field and Morse (1985).
- The study aim was stated in an honest and open manner and the involvement required from the participants made explicit.

I noted recently (Ford, 1994) that the participants within Ford's study chose to be identified and were proud of, and owned their experiences. For me this showed real collaboration with participants and a mutuality truly reflecting phenomenological assumptions.

Sample size

Although the findings when random sampling is used may be considered to be more representative and therefore more generalizable (Polit and Hungler, 1987), random sampling does not guarantee that the phenomena to be explored are evenly distributed within the final sample (Field and Morse, 1985). I chose purposive sampling to guide my selection of participants in this study. This approach allowed the selection of a sample of people who 'represent' the phenomenon in question so that the findings can include as much of the phenomenon as possible (Polit and Hungler, 1987). The number of interviews conducted in a phenomenological study is also less important than the extent to which the phenomenon is explored in each interview (Drew, 1989). At the time of the study, I understood that the size of the sample and the nature of the study made generalization of the results improbable (Field and Morse, 1985). However, I now believe this to be untrue. I was also aware of the potential of my own conscious bias in the choice of the sample as this was also one of convenience, but did not consider this of import.

Data gathering strategies

It is worth noting at this point that the exploratory and investigative nature of data gathering and analysis are in reality more interwoven and simultaneously undertaken than my neat separation suggests. This ensures clarity and is frequently a requirement of examining authorities, if the research represents coursework.

Phenomenological methodology described by Colaizzi (1978) provided a framework for the collection and analysis of data. According to Omery (1983), Colaizzi (1978) advises that the data collection and analysis should occur simultaneously. He also stresses the importance of describing in detail the data collection methods. In view of the subjective nature of the data, I have tried to quote directly the words of the participants.

From a phenomenological perspective, it would be appropriate to think of the data gathering part of the process as the educational development of the researcher. The researcher is finding ways to develop a deeper understanding of the phenomenon being investigated. Phenomenologists educate themselves in two ways: fieldwork education; which may consist of transcribed taped conversations, interviewing, observing, talking with participants, case studies, diaries and written accounts; and reading. Material that may yield significant understanding to enhance this education can be gained from a variety of sources. Van Manen (1984) suggests the researchers' own personal experience, the experience of others, biographies, reconstructed life stories, novels containing vivid description, and other artistic and literary sources. I chose to enhance my fieldwork education using written accounts of the experience and by interviews.

Written account

As we ask what it is like, in order to remain close to the experience, it may be helpful to stay very concrete, to ask the person to think of, or to focus on, a specific instant, situation, person, or event. Thus the whole event can be explored to the fullest. I asked two groups of ENB 998 students, totalling 30 in number, to complete a written account. The written information was requested in two parts. Part one asked for demographic data from the participants, in order to build a career profile, and part two asked an open question related to their perceptions and experience. The open question asked them to:

> Focus on a recent high quality classroom session in which you learnt. *What was important to you* in that session which made it high quality?
> Please give details and examples where possible.

I could also have asked the participants to write a direct account of a personal experience as they lived through it, or another open request. In the open question which asked for thoughts and perceptions of participants on high quality education, I refrained from giving any definition or meaning of quality education, inviting participants to respond as they chose. This allowed the participant to define their own frame of reference (Barker, 1991) and limited my bias.

Some descriptions were richer than others, just as in everyday life we learn more from some people than others, however, there was always something of value. Sometimes it is easier to talk than to write about an experience, because writing forces us into a more reflective attitude which may make it more difficult to stay close to the experience as it is immediately lived.

Interviews

As with all naturalistic research, the researcher must build a trusting relationship with the respondent in order to engage in cooperative dialogue. This is particularly so with phenomenological research. The point of phenomenological research is to borrow other people's experiences, and their reflections on their experiences, in order to be better able to come to an understanding of the deeper meaning of, or significance of, an aspect of human experience, in the context of the whole of the human experience. As the aim of the research is to delve into the experience, and this will often involve strong feelings, the participants must be able to speak with ease, to understand and express inner feelings and express the experiences that accompany these feelings (Omery, 1983). This requires good listening skills, being able spontaneously to encourage people to describe aspects of their experience they normally ignore without leading them, and being able to verify with the participant that the meaning of the experience has been properly understood. It may also require the presence of a counsellor as feelings are uncovered, exposed and examined.

One of the greatest values of the interview in relation to experience is that it allows both parties to explore the meaning of the questions and answers involved. Areas of uncertainty or ambiguity can be clarified instantly, to avoid misinterpretation (Brenner *et al.*, 1985). During an interview, immediate responses are given to questions which deal with different levels of detail and complexity, and a more flexible, in-depth and richer source of data is provided through these personal accounts (Cohen and Manion, 1989).

I conducted a total of five semi-structured interviews, selecting from the participants who indicated on their written account that they were willing to be interviewed. Because the interviewees are few in number, to maintain their anonymity and confidentiality, their career profile was included within the whole sample group. Participants were contacted by telephone and appointments scheduled for a time and venue convenient to them. I tried to minimize the likelihood of interruptions and chose seating arrangements that facilitated verbal interaction without, I hope, appearing threatening to the participant (Hargie *et al.*, 1981). During a research interview, the interviewer should be able to show attentiveness: listening actively to what is being said, sitting at an appropriate distance and adopting a posture which suggests a relaxed manner and openness to the information that the participant is willing to share (Barker, 1991).

I tried to reassure the participants, and felt I succeeded in creating a relaxed atmosphere. I maintained eye contact appropriate to deep conversation (Hargie *et al.*, 1981). Barker (1991) suggests that the quality of information generated in an interview is entirely dependent on the interviewer's behaviour. I commenced by reiterating issues of confidentiality and then progressed to the purpose of the interview. Each interviewee was given the opportunity to read through their written account and indicate whether it reflected what they intended it to. I informed each interviewee why they specifically had been selected, how the interview would proceed, and the maximum time it could take. This set the agenda for the interviews (Barker, 1991). I invited any questions at this stage before proceeding. All interviews were recorded using an audio-cassette tape-recorder to ensure accurate data collection and to allow ease of rechecking information (Bogdan and Taylor, 1984). A maximum of 45 minutes was allocated for each interview, and each interview was transcribed in full. Transcription is a lengthy and laborious task, however, data analysis cannot proceed without it in phenomenology. It is important to analyse all the data, not simply that which meets the researcher's needs. There are no short cuts.

To assist in focusing each interview, I prepared an interview guide; for me this was based on the preliminary analysis of the interviewee's written account. This remained secondary to any opportunities that arose to explore beyond this guide, as long as the discussion remained within the parameters of the overall research.

I began with the following opening sentence:

> I'm interested in what constitutes high quality classroom education, in which learning takes place. The things I would like us to talk about from your own experience are:

I used an interview guide for all interviews to maintain a balance in structure, as I wished to include those areas I thought to be important to clarify, while enhancing the interviewee's scope for introducing topics that they considered relevant and important (Bogdan and Taylor, 1984). This also served as an aide memoire.

Often it is not necessary to ask too many questions. Patience or silence is a more tactful way of prompting. If there seems to be a thought block, the last sentence or idea can be repeated in a questioning tone. If the participant begins to generalize or opinionate about the experience, a way of turning the discourse back to the level of lived experience is to ask for an example.

Data gathering such as this allows the researcher to become better informed, and enriched by this experience, to be more able to render the full significance of meaning.

I was aware with these participants of bias, the need of the interviewee to please the interviewer, and the potential of myself as interviewer to seek out answers and information that supported my preconceived ideas (Field and Morse, 1985). Immediately following each interview, fieldnotes were made on the ease of interaction, non-verbal communication, and the subjective impressions of the interview to aid my reflections on the process.

The phenomenological style selected at the outset of the study serves as the framework for a step-by-step process of data analysis. Colaizzi's eight steps from data analysis are given as one example (Figure 7.4), which I used to structure data analysis. I believe data analysis to be a strength of my study and, as a result, greater attention is given to this.

As the primary task of data analysis is to reveal the meaning of an event, the descriptions must be in terms of the meaning it has for the participants. The task of coding the transcriptions and developing themes and categories representing increasing levels of abstraction, takes susbstantial amounts of time to complete. Additionally, this method requires time to develop the initial coding decisions, to become immersed in the data, and to complete the analysis process. The data are then described in the natural and unique

1. Read through the entire protocol (the subject's description) for a sense of the whole. Taped interviews need to be listened to, and be transcribed verbatum.

2. Extract significant statements that directly pertain to the investigated topic.

3. Formulate the significant statements into more general restatements.

4. Formulate meanings as they emerge from the significant statements. This involves creative insight, which remains faithful to the original data. Validation can be achieved by returning the data to the research participants or to 'judges'.

5. Repeat the above steps for each protocol and organize the formulated meanings into themes, theme clusters and categories.
    (a) Validate the themes, theme clusters and categories by referring back to the original protocols to see if any data have been ignored or added to.
    (b) If there are contradictions, this may be the real and valid experience. These data should not be ignored or discarded.

6. The results of the analysis so far are then integrated into an exhaustive description of the investigated topic.

7. Formulate the exhaustive description of the phenomenon into a statement of identification of its fundamental structure.

8. To validate the analysis, return to each participant (co-researcher) and ask if this analysis describes their experience. If the participant/co-researcher adds or deletes any information, incorporate these new data into the final product.

Figure 7.4 Data analysis using the eight steps advocated by Colaizzi (1978)

language of the event. This serves to highlight the need for time to complete a study of this nature, but also the rigour of the method.

Profile of participants

Just as in a novel, vivid description brings the characters to life, the participants in a phenomenological study may be enlivened by a career profile or pen portrait. I chose to use a career profile of the participants to highlight who they were as a group of nurses. Ford (1994) used stunning pen portraits accompanied by photographs to create empathy with her participants. This, I believe, reinforces the person-centredness of the approach and further entices the reader into the research question.

Exploration and analysis of the data

Data are explored and analysed using the steps of Colaizzi's (1978) phenomenological approach to data collection, which uses thematic analysis. Aspects of Burnard's (1991) method of analysing interview transcripts were also incorporated. There appeared to be many different approaches to handling the data, with similar processes involved, and analysis taking place within a structured framework. I chose the Colaizzi (1978) method as this seemed a logical and step-by-step approach for the novice.

Step 1

All the written accounts and transcripts were carefully and thoughtfully read to gain a 'feeling for them; a making sense out of them' (Colaizzi, 1978). The aim was to become immersed in the data, more fully aware, and to enter the other person's frame of reference (Rogers, 1951).

Step 2

Multiple photocopies of the written accounts and the transcripts were made. The copies were essential to make extractions while retaining a sense of context. Significant statements and phrases pertaining to High Quality Education in the Classroom were then extracted, cut from the photocopied written accounts and the transcripts, and also made into a complete list.

At times it was difficult to extract significant statements or phrases as these were interwoven with the session titles. I did not want to reveal the session titles as this would, in turn, reveal which of my lecturer colleague's sessions were regarded as High Quality sessions. More specifically, it would reveal whose sessions had been omitted, and I assumed that these had not been regarded as High Quality sessions. I felt that to focus the participant's attention on an example, when completing the written account, would be valuable in revealing more specific detail, which it was. However, at times, this increased the difficulty in extrapolating the significant statements or phrases.

While Colaizzi (1978) advocates examining for minutiae in the significant statements and phrases, I felt unable to follow in this way for two reasons. First, I was aware of the time-line that I intended to follow for this research, however constraintive it became. Secondly, as a novice researcher, I wanted to guard against losing the sense of context and the relative importance of issues.

For example, one statement read:

> The session allowed us to explore different teaching methods – some commonly used, some more obscure, and to experience the pros and cons of these methods within the classroom.

I felt that this statement related to teaching methods, however, if desired, it could have been further reduced to include: exploring, teaching methods, common teaching methods, obscure teaching methods, pros of teaching methods and cons of teaching methods. By further dividing the statement in this way, I would have lost the meaning of high quality education in the classroom in the statement.

The significant statements still amounted to 174 and as such cannot be detailed in full. A vast amount of data were generated. A phrase which seems unimportant initially, after reading and re-reading the interview transcripts, what may have been overlooked could be one of the most important data items.

A selection of statements now follow, which I have chosen to represent the variety of responses given by the participants, and to give a flavour of the content of the study:

> I feel that the important factors that contribute to high quality sessions include a teacher who involves the class in participation . . .

> I found it of significance to me for career development

> A high quality session is one that leaves the learner wanting to know more of the subject of the session

> The tutor was friendly and appeared approachable

> I also found separating into small groups for a brainstorm good as this broke up the session and made it varied

> the classroom sessions made me feel comfortable as the atmosphere was relaxed . . . and the group supportive and friendly

> The handouts were also very useful

The extracted statements were identified noting the code number of the participant, and the sequence of each excerpt within the original written account and/or the interview transcript.

The 'dross' was discarded. Field and Morse (1985) use the term dross to denote the unusable part of an interview, the issues that are unrelated to the research in general terms.

Examples of the data that I considered to be dross from both the written accounts and interviews were:

> The session was the one on . . . (title given)
> The title of the lesson was . . . (title given)

There was very little of the data that could be termed dross. The significant statements and phrases should, and did, account for almost all of the written account and interview data (Burnard, 1991).

Steps 3 and 4

Meanings were formulated from the significant statements. The statements were read repeatedly, reviewed in relation to their sequence in the transcript, reflected upon, and the meaning of the excerpt identified. Creative insight was needed at this stage to move away from what the participants said, to what they meant, while still remaining faithful to the original data (Colaizzi, 1978).

The formulation of meanings, I feel, was an easier part of the data analysis. As my clinical background was in intensive care nursing with children, I have learnt, and practised, constant interpretation of the meaning of data throughout my career. I recognized that this data analysis and interpretation was different, but the principles appeared to be very similar with some reliance on intuitive and gut feeling. The tapes were constantly replayed and the written accounts re-read to facilitate the interpretation of data.

Step 5

Formulated meanings were then organized into Themes. Phenomenological Themes are the structures of experience. When a phenomenon is analysed, we are trying to determine what the themes are, that is, the structures that make up the experience. Van Manen (1984) suggests two approaches to identifying themes. One is to highlight emergent themes by asking what statements or phrases seem particularly revealing about the experience being described, and the other is to take a line-by-line approach identifying in each sentence what this sentence tells us about the experience.

To me as a novice, this task initially felt monumentous, however, I was soon able to recognize repeated words, phrases and concepts. Having noted this, some of the phrases did not fall easily into one Theme, for example, one statement read:

> Everyone in the room was offering their full participation as it was a very realistic and well interpreted subject.

I felt that this statement could have been analysed within the Themes of Group Participation, The Subject, The Lecturer (who interpreted the subject), or Teaching Methods (by which the students' participation was facilitated). As a result I placed this and other statements and phrases into multiple Themes

Approaching the data in this way, I hoped to isolate topics which did not overlap and that made the data more manageable, however, I was also conscious that the themes did not do justice to the richness of the phenomena. A theme simply alludes to, or hints at, one aspect of the phenomenon (van Manen, 1984). The Themes headed A4 size sheets of paper, and relevant statements cut from the written accounts and interview transcripts were then affixed to appropriate sheets with a Theme heading. Each of the Themes was allocated a specific colour of highlighter pen and colour coded to facilitate ease of identification, when referring back to the original statements (Burnard, 1991).

There were 30 initial themes concerning High Quality Education in the Classroom, which are shown in Figure 7.5. A4 sheets with Theme headings were grouped together, thus I noted that as themes recurred, commonality existed in the descriptions I was gathering. The Themes were grouped and evolved into Theme Clusters, which are shown in Figure 7.6. Clusters of Themes were validated by referring back to the written accounts and audiotape transcripts to check that none of the data had been ignored or added to. If contradictory Themes emerge, this may be the real and valid experience, which should not be ignored or discarded (Colaizzi, 1978). All themes were retained and no contradictions were evident.

The way in which I grouped the Themes concerning High Quality Education in the Classroom into Theme Clusters concerning High Quality Education in the Classroom is shown in Figure 7.7.

Eventually, Theme Categories concerning High Quality Education in the Classroom were formed from the reduced Theme Clusters, as shown in Figure 7.8. Selected participants were asked to check the appropriateness or otherwise of the category system by looking at their written account and interview transcript.

- Evaluation
- The environment
- Group participation
- Students motivating themselves
- Psychological safety
- Career development
- Knowledgeable lecturer
- Enthusiastic lecturer
- Well planned session
- Choice of teaching method
- Lecturer as motivator
- Research based session
- Time to reflect
- Learning from each other
- Feelings
- Handout/references
- Individual exercises
- Summary at end
- Stated objectives
- Adult approach
- New knowledge
- Hypothetical situations
- Interested lecturer
- Applicable subject
- Relevance to course
- Supportive lecturer
- Skilled lecturer
- Valued students
- Audio-visual aids
- Resources

Figure 7.5 The themes that emerged from participants concerning high quality education in the classroom

- Motivation
- The student group
- The subject
- Psychological safety
- The lecturer
- Overall organization of the session
- Teaching methods/group participation
- Feelings

Figure 7.6 The theme clusters that emerged from student participants concerning high quality education in the classroom

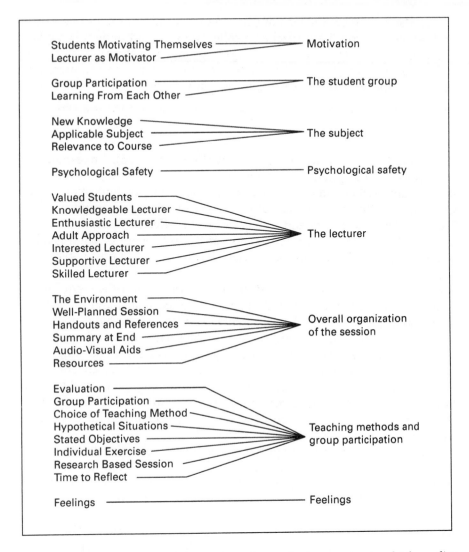

Students Motivating Themselves ──────── Motivation
Lecturer as Motivator ───

Group Participation ─────── The student group
Learning From Each Other ───

New Knowledge ───
Applicable Subject ─── The subject
Relevance to Course ───

Psychological Safety ──────── Psychological safety

Valued Students ───
Knowledgeable Lecturer ───
Enthusiastic Lecturer ───
Adult Approach ─── The lecturer
Interested Lecturer ───
Supportive Lecturer ───
Skilled Lecturer ───

The Environment ───
Well-Planned Session ───
Handouts and References ─── Overall organization
Summary at End ─── of the session
Audio-Visual Aids ───
Resources ───

Evaluation ───
Group Participation ───
Choice of Teaching Method ───
Hypothetical Situations ─── Teaching methods and
Stated Objectives ─── group participation
Individual Exercise ───
Research Based Session ───
Time to Reflect ───

Feelings ──────── Feelings

Figure 7.7 The grouping of themes into theme clusters concerning high quality education in the classroom

```
●  Issues relating to the students
●  Issues relating to the lecturer
```

Figure 7.8 Theme categories that emerged from student participants concerning high quality education in the classroom

This also provided a means of verifying the validity of my categorizing process. In addition, I approached a colleague who had undertaken qualitative research to scrutinize the emergent themes and theme clusters. The colleague brought forward similar themes and clusters to my own, and because of the similarity, I elected to remain with my own.

Step 6

Following the procedure advocated by Colaizzi (1978), an exhaustive description of the phenomenon was written. This was formulated from the student participants' own words on High Quality Education in the Classroom, with my own narrative for clarification and emphasis. The Themes, Theme Clusters and Categories were reflected upon to further a sense of the whole of the phenomenon of the experience of High Quality Education in the Classroom, as described by students on a post-registration course.

I chose to structure my exhaustive description around the eight Theme Clusters. I felt that the 30 initial Themes were too many, and unmanageable. This approach would have presented a 'micro' view, that is, too many small Themes with little depth or detail. Alternatively, to interpret data based on the two final emergent Theme Categories of 'Issues Relating to the Lecturer' and 'Issues Relating to the Student' would have constituted a 'macro' view. There would have been much depth and detail, and I would have found difficulty maintaining a logical and comprehensible structure in the description. Theme Clusters concerning High Quality in the Classroom therefore provided a manageable framework.

A judgement of relative importance was made according to the size of the Theme Clusters, that is the number of student participants who made statements and phrases relating to those issues, and also the frequency of actual statements. The two Theme Clusters of Psychological Safety and Feelings were included for different reasons. Although the frequency of participants who discussed these issues was limited, I decided their meanings were important enough to me as a teacher to warrant inclusion. The emphasis lay in the strength of feeling that emerged and the significance of the meaning.

An extract of the exhaustive description now follows as word limitation prevents inclusion of the whole:

> Psychological safety is of utmost importance in the classroom. Those students who discussed this stated that they felt potentially vulnerable in an unknown group. One student commented:
>
>> I feel group work allows the less assertive student to express ideas of their own in smaller groups, therefore feeling less intimidated if they make a wrong suggestion.

The approach of the lecturer is an important contribution in creating a psychologically safe environment, as revealed:

> The lecturer was very open and the class was made to feel that any point that they had to share was important, and at no time incorrect.

Other student participants said that they felt able and secure enough to ask questions and have them answered.

The atmosphere created also positively influenced the outcome of learning:

> the atmosphere was relaxed and informal. It didn't feel like learning, more like sharing ideas.

Copies of the original interview transcripts were kept at hand during the writing up process, as were the A4 sheets with the colour-coded statements. The constant referral back to the original work ensures that the researcher stays close to the original meanings and contexts (Burnard, 1991). The description of the phenomenon enables a deeper understanding of the student's perception of high quality education in the classroom.

Step 7

From the description of the phenomenon of High Quality Education in the Classroom given by the participating students, I could then formulate my description of the essential structure of High Quality Education in the Classroom. This involved putting aside the participants' comments, then reflecting to enable me to write a complete description, a story, which was my own interpretation in my own words.

Step 8

To validate the data analysis, Colaizzi (1978) suggests that the researcher returns to each participant to verify that the essential structure describes their experience. If the participant adds or deletes any information, this is incorporated into the final product.

Phenomenological writing

Phenomenological research aims to illuminate the features of a lived experience that make it visible. Every phenomenological study is therefore only one person's interpretation of that lived experience; it is an example. A phenomenological description describes an original, of which the description is only an example. If the description is powerful, then it allows the reader to see the deeper meaning of the lived experience it describes.

It is a function of the appropriateness of the themes and the degree of thoughtfulness that the descriptions can be captured. A description is a good one if it reawakens our experience of the phenomenon it describes in such a manner that we experience the more foundational grounds of the experience (van Manen, 1984).

Language is a central concern in phenomenological research because responsive–reflective writing is essential to phenomenology. It involves the total physical and mental being, and to write phenomenologically is the untiring effort to write a sensitive grasp of being itself.

When writing the research report, incorporating the literature can prove demanding. A literature review is considered inappropriate in the initial stages of a phenomenological study (Field and Morse, 1985), however, if the study is undertaken as part of a course requirement, the examining body may require it. More usually the literature is chosen which supports the findings, and may be included, at Step Six of the data analysis, or within the discussion of the findings. What must be remembered is that the level of analysis within the discussion of the literature should be equitable to a literature review, however it is integrated within the research.

The purpose of the literature is to continue the educational process undertaken by the researcher during data gathering. Many examples of good practice are available to the reader for inspiration when undertaking this sometimes daunting task (Haase, 1987; Girot, 1993; Morse *et al.*, 1994). Phenomenology is an appropriate methodology for exploring those areas where little literature exists.

Findings

Van Manen (1984) remarked that, as in poetry, it is inappropriate to ask for or expect a summary or conclusion. To summarize in order to present the result would be destructive, as the poem is the result. The poem is the thing, as the essential structure is the thing.

The outcome of the research process is a description of the structure of the phenomenon under study. An advantage of using this method is the richness of the data gathered, knowing that the deepest understanding of the structure of the experience has been discovered. The phenomenological method allows for recognition of another as a unique individual with a unique set of experiences (Watson, 1988), but also allows the researcher an opportunity to gain insight into the self. Awareness of the researcher's own intuitive caring nature empowers a response of increased understanding when the phenomenon is encountered in the future (Pallikkathayil and Morgan, 1991).

Methodological rigour

The rigour of phenomenology, as a method of understanding, is the refusal to accept a perception without first examining the influence of underlying beliefs naively held by the perceiver (Drew, 1989). The phenomenological researcher refuses to ground a study in unexamined beliefs, to start from a point of trust or reliance in the validity of commonsense understanding. Phenomenological research recognizes, identifies and incorporates where appropriate the biases of the researcher (Omery, 1983). Researchers study issues that are important to them, and about which they care, sometimes passionately. Validity is established by returning to the participants with the data. Alternatively, or, in addition, 'research judges' may be used to verify the categories that emerge from the data. This dual approach was used in my own research, however, this may prove difficult. The participants may not yet be ready to look back on their interview data, particularly if this represented discussing a sensitive or traumatic experience for them. This may have been an issue faced by Williams (1993) when exploring stress in the paediatric intensive care unit from the fathers' perspective. Rigour is also achieved by bracketing. In my research, this occurred both at the outset of the process by completing a written account, and throughout, by the use of a reflective diary.

Phenomenology does not expect duplicate behaviour from duplicate data. Duplication may occur when the meanings of experiences are similar, and generalizations may be made based on these similar meanings. Exact duplication is not required (Omery, 1983). In addition, lack of acceptance for the methodology also leads some phenomenological researchers to dwell on issues of validity and reliability rather than focusing on the valuable knowledge generated by this method (Salsberry, 1989).

From a first-time novice researcher with a reluctance to undertake any research methodology, I have developed an enthusiastic interest in the phenomenological perspective. From formulating the research question and becoming immersed in the data, I progressed to a point of virtual obsession during data analysis.

Conclusion

I believe that to undertake phenomenological research successfully, the researcher must share the assumptions of phenomenological philosophy which underpin the method. Within my more recent experience of supervising phenomenological research studies, I have observed those who I believe to have personal philosophies that share more with positivism, undertaking phenomenological research. This is done with vigorous attention to formal stages and driving the data towards unnatural methodological perfection. This lies in opposition to true phenomenology.

Currently, phenomenology struggles to be accepted as a valid method of theory development. This may be due to few nurse researchers being prepared and experienced in this methodology, also a problem identified during supervision. The lack of external funding for phenomenological studies also presents difficulties (Pallikkathayil and Morgan, 1991).

Husserl (1931, cited in Drew, 1989) spoke of the danger of discounting lived experience and human subjectivity. The danger of which he warned is that when the subjective is devalued or ignored, we can become removed from experience as it is lived, losing touch with our feelings, and the feelings of those around us. We then lose understanding and eventual meaning. Feelings are our first response to a situation or problem, and therefore should be taken into account by researchers. By striving to 'see' and to describe experience, phenomenological researchers hope to draw thinking more closely to experiencing: to make concepts more accurate, more precise, and closer to the reality of experience (Oiler and Boyd, 1989). The phenomenological method is promoted therefore as essential to theory development in the humanistic discipline of nursing.

References

Appleton C (1993) The art of nursing: the experience of patients and nurses. *Journal of Advanced Nursing* 18, 892–9.

Barker P J (1991) The Questionnaire. In Cormack D F S (Ed.) *The Research Process in Nursing*. Blackwell Scientific Publications, Oxford.

Beck C T (1992) The lived experience of postpartum depression: a phenomenological study. *Nursing Research* 41 (3), 166–70.

Benner P (1985) Quality of life: a phenomenological perspective on explanation, prediction and understanding. *Advances in Nursing Science* 8, 1–14.

Bennett L (1991) Adolescent girls' experience of marital violence: a phenomenolgoical study. *Journal of Advanced Nursing* 16, 431–38.

Bogdan R and Taylor S (1984) *Introduction to Qualitative Research Methods*, 2nd edn. Wiley, New York.

Boud, D, Keogh, R and Walker, D (1985) *Reflection: Turning Experience into Learning*. Kogan Page, London.

Brenner M, Brown J and Canter D (Eds) (1985) *The Research Interview, Uses and Approaches*. Academic Press, London.

Burnard, P and Morrison, P (1990) *Nursing Research in Action: Developing Basic Skills*. Macmillan, London.

Burnard P (1991) A method of analysing interview transcripts in qualitative research. *Nurse Education Today* 11, 461–6.

Cohen M Z (1987) A historical overview of the phenomenologic movement. *IMAGE: Journal of Nursing Scholarship* 19 (1), 31–4.

Cohen L and Manion L (1989) *Research Methods in Education*, 3rd edn. Routledge, London.

Colaizzi P (1978) Psychological research as the phenomenologists view it. In Valle R and King M (Eds) *Existential Phenomenological Alternatives For Psychology*. Oxford University Press, New York.

Drew, N. (1989) The interviewer's experience as data in phenomenological research. *Western Journal of Nursing Research* 11 (4), 431–9.

Field, P A and Morse J M (1985) *Nursing Research: The Application of Qualitative Approaches.* Croom Helm, London.

Ford P (1994) What older people, as patients in continuing care, value in nurses. Unpublished Masters Thesis, Keele University.

Gadamer H G (1975) *Truth and Method.* Seabury Press, New York.

Giorgi A (1970) *Psychology as a Human Science: A Phenomenologically Based Approach.* Harper & Row, New York.

Girot E (1993) Assessment of competence in clinical practice: a phenomenological approach. *Journal of Advanced Nursing* 18, 114–19.

Haase J E (1987) Components of courage in chronically ill adolescents: a phenomenological study. *Advances in Nursing Science* 9 (2), 64–80.

Hargie O, Saunders C and Dickson D (1981) *Social Skills in Interpersonal Communication.* Croom Helm, London.

James N (1992) A postscript to nursing. In Abbott A and Sapsford R (Eds) *Research into Practice: A Reader for Nurses and the Caring Professions.* Open University Press, Milton Keynes.

Leininger M (1985) *Qualitative Research Methods in Nursing.* Grune & Stratton, New York.

Lynch-Sauer, J (1985) Using a phenomenological research method to study nursing phenomena. In Leininger M M (Ed.) *Qualitative Research Methods in Nursing.* Grune & Stratton, New York.

van Manen N (1984) Practising phenomenological writing. *Phenomenology and Pedagogy* 2 (1), 36–69.

Merleau-Ponty, M (1962) *Phenomenology of Perception.* Routledge and Kegan Paul, London.

Merleau-Ponty M (1964) *The Primacy of Perception.* Northwestern University Press, Evanston.

Morse J M, Bottorff J L and Hutchinson S (1994) The phenomenology of comfort. *Journal of Advanced Nursing* 20, 189–95.

Munhall P L and Oiler C (1986) *Nursing Research: A Qualitative Perspective.* Appleton-Century-Crofts, Norwalk, CT.

National Boards for England and Wales (1985) *Teaching and Assessing in Clinical Practice Number 998 – Outline Curricula.* The National Boards for England and Wales, London.

Oiler C (1982) The phenomenological approach in nursing research. *Nursing Research* 31 (3), 178–81.

Oiler C and Boyd C (1989) Phenomenological research in nursing: clarifying the issues. *Nursing Science Quarterly* 2 (1), 16–19.

Omery A (1983) Phenomenology: a method for nursing research. *Advances in Nursing Science* 6 (2), 49–63.

Pallikkathayil L and Morgan S A (1991) Phenomenology as a method for conducting clinical research. *Applied Nursing Research* 4 (4), 195–99.

Parse R R (1981) The experience of laughter: a phenomenological study. *Nursing Science Quarterly* 6 (1), 39–43.

Parse R R, Coyne A B and Smith M J (1986) Nursing research: qualitative methods. *Nursing Science Quarterly* 1, 86–90.

Patton M G (1980) *Qualitative Evaluation Methods.* Sage Publications, California.

Polit D F and Hungler B P (1987) *Nursing Research, Principles and Methods*, 3rd edn. Lippincott, Philadelphia.

Reason P and Rowan J (Eds) (1981) *Human Inquiry, a Sourcebook of New Paradigm Research*. Wiley, Chichester.

Rogers C R (1951) *Client Centred Therapy*. Constable, London.

Salsberry P J (1989) Phenomenological research in nursing: commentary and responses. *Nursing Science Quarterly* 2 (1), 9–13.

Spiegelberg H. (1960) *The Phenomenological Movement*, Vol. 1. Martinus Nijoff, Hague.

Swanson-Kauffman K and Schonwald E (1988) Phenomenology. In Sarter B (Ed.) *Paths to Knowledge: Innovative Research Methods for Nursing*. National League for Nursing, New York.

Van Kaam, A (1959) Phenomenological analysis: exemplified by a study of the experience of really being understood. *Individual Psychology* 15, 66–72.

Van Kaam A (1966) *Existential Foundations of Psychology*, Vol. 3. Duguesna University Press, Pittsburgh.

Watson J (1988) *Nursing: Human Science and Human Care. A Theory of Nursing*. Appleton-Century-Crofts, Norwalk, CT.

Webb C (1992) The use of the first person in academic writing: objectivity, language and gatekeeping. *Journal of Advanced Nursing* 17 (5), 747–52.

Williams C A (1993) The phenomenon of stress in the paediatric intensive care unit: the fathers' perspective. Unpublished Undergraduate Thesis, Manchester University.

8

Triangulation: an issue of method mixing

Jayne Beeby

The second chapter on phenomenology demonstrates how theoretical concepts can be broadly interpreted and applied in contrasting ways to the practice of research. While the value system underpinning this approach appears similar to the previous chapter this account explores and uses phenomenology in a positivist way:

- *the impetus for this study is unusual;*
- *triangulation – a difficult concept is explored in its various forms and applied to this study;*
- *data analysis provides a useful cross-reference and complement to Chapter 7.*

The purpose of this chapter is to share my experience of designing and then implementing a research study. I hope to share the insights I gained from attempting to apply the concept of 'triangulation' to the practice of 'doing research', thus highlighting a paradox between the success of testing theory and the failure of losing data while being true to the methodology chosen to complete my study.

I would say that my experience of using the research process would be that of the novice. The experience I will be sharing is that gained from completing a research project for an undergraduate programme of study. Prior to that I had, in my teaching role, been running a English National Board long course which valued the use of applying research to clinical practice. This was achieved by teaching others about the research process and developing their critical–thinking skills in questioning research reports in a variety of ways. My interest in research began from the delivery of the curriculum in relation to my own area of clinical expertise, that of intensive care nursing. I was both frightened and excited by the idea of completing a 'proper' research study. Questions of 'Could I do it?' 'Do I understand enough?' 'What should I research?' all came to mind.

While the project was part of an assessment programme I was undertaking, it would provide me with first-hand experience of the research process. I was excited because I wanted my work to mean something, not just to myself, but to others in my field of expertise. Not only would I know about the research process, I would begin to understand the practicalities of doing research. I place highly in my style of teaching the ability to role model practice, this I believe strongly influences learning and socializes students into an expected way of being. Understanding the processes of research I hoped would encourage me to share a realistic view of research process with my students, motivating them to think in a questioning way and begin to develop their own skills in exploring and testing their ideas. The research project itself was supported by a year's research methods course which developed a foundation of knowledge that provided the basis for much of the decision making involved in implementing the research process. My first area of angst was which subject? I knew that this would be a major piece of work to complete and I felt that I would need a subject which would help motivate me, even when the 'going got tough'. I found my subject inadvertently one day when nursing rather than teaching.

The origins of my research study were rooted in a clinical incident which occurred to me during a morning shift on duty concerning a lady known for this chapter as 'Flo'. This incident was representative of my thoughts at that time in relation to a dilemma I was beginning to question of technology versus humanism and the position of caring in that dilemma.

'Flo'

My interest in the phenomenon of caring developed from one particular incident in my nursing practice in the intensive care unit (ITU). I went to work on an early duty, which started at 7 am, where I was allocated to nurse Flo for the shift. She was critically ill, being nursed in the side-room, and had developed severe peritonitis following major bowel surgery. At that point Flo had an open abdominal wound and was returning daily to theatres for abdominal lavages. Flo was being supported with 'the works'. This meant that Flo was being supported by all the technical aspects of care prevalent in ITU, such as the ventilator, haemodynamic monitoring, inotropic support, etc. The ITU had been especially busy during the night and as always the complement of staff had been supplemented with agency nurses to provide the additional cover needed. I took over from the night nurse who looked tired and hassled. Between the hours of 7 am and 11 am, I checked the equipment, carried out my observations, cleaned the room, took away the dirty equipment and rubbish, stocked up the room with all that was needed for the day, and attended to four sets of doctors, each reviewing Flo's condition. Finally at 11 am while completing the hourly observations I began to take notice of Flo, her face was grimaced, although heavily sedated she appeared to be trying to speak. After struggling to understand her several attempts to speak with an endotracheal tube in her mouth I finally got the message, 'I've had enough, I want this to stop, I want to die, let me go, why don't you let me go?' I was floored. Needless to say, I stood back feeling awful. Flo had needed to say this all morning and I had been too busy to listen to her need. What happened to caring?

My views

Since my experience with Flo, I have given the idea of caring much thought. Caring, in my nursing practice in intensive care, values the relationship that the patient and nurse find themselves in. The quality and depth of that relationship is both unequal and unpredictable; the patient is often critically ill, their condition unstable and by the nature of the situation, completely dependent. Therefore the patient is completely reliant upon the nurse. Caring for someone requires highly specialized interpersonal and technical skills, the person receiving care must not be forgotten. The nurse when caring must show sensitivity when communicating with the patient, and soften the effects of the intensive care environment. The technology is there as an adjunct to care, not to do the caring for the nurse. The nurse must respect the person's integrity, caring for the whole person, he or she is the patient's advocate: their eyes, ears and voice. The nurse is in the position to make the experience of being in intensive care a humane one, which values the needs and wishes of the patient and family. The incident with Flo challenged my beliefs, as I had acted in response to the rites of practice arising from the environment rather than responding to the needs of the person. Which should take precedence? The competing tensions of underlying beliefs within myself and within my workplace were causing conflict and I began to wonder if other nurses in intensive care had considered what caring was for them in this type of clinical environment.

To begin to find answers to my questions it was the purpose of my study to describe the meaning of caring for nurses practising within the intensive care setting. For myself I began to recognize that the technological innovations being utilized and the attitude in which they had been used encouraged a 'particularistic' way of practising nursing, focusing on different parts of care rather than considering the impact the whole situation may have on a person. The rites of practice in this environment were underpinned by a belief system grounded in reductionism which challenged my own beliefs related to humanism and holism.

Qualitative methods

The nature of my research question sought to understand caring, from the perspective of those who experience caring, making implicit knowledge explicit (Field and Morse, 1985). Therefore to answer the research question a minimum of structure, imposed by the research design, was necessary to understand the experience of others. I therefore felt that qualitative methods were the more appropriate to use. Reason and Rowan (1981) argue the point that researchers should utilize research methods which are representative of their personal beliefs and value system. This they suggest increases the researcher's level of motivation and interest in completing a research study. Moccia (1988) concurs with this view and believes that nurses should choose research activities that reflect their own philosophy and world-view of nursing. Nursing for me is a dynamic and complex process, which cannot be reduced to a number of measurable parts. Caring is a part of that process. Individuals bring to any situation a uniqueness which can only be ascribed to the wholeness of themselves. I wanted to access the 'wealth of rich data of a softer nature', arising from experience (Melia, 1982, p. 328), to explain and understand the complexity of caring in the intensive care unit. Using a paradigm that enabled congruence with my values further influenced my choice in using a qualitative research design. A qualitative approach would enable me to look at caring in the context of the intensive care environment but more importantly understand the meaning of care for those involved in the nurse–patient relationship. I not only would be able to value the whole person, but also value the uniqueness of their experience. With these points in mind I chose phenomenology as the research methodology to underpin my study.

Phenomenology

Phenomenological enquiry is said to begin in silence (Spiegelberg, 1976). When using phenomenology this is the beginning of a process described as bracketing (Oiler, 1982; Omery, 1983; Swanson-Kauffman and Schonwald, 1988; Drew, 1989). This process does not eliminate my perspective, but by reflecting on the phenomenon in question, i.e. caring, brings it into view, allowing the researcher's perspective to be understood and valued within the research process.

   Phenomenology is a research method grounded in philosophy. The value of phenomenology arose from the failure of natural science to value a person's subjective reality by predicting and controlling behaviour, which Omery (1983) believes developed a view of man which was simplistic and demeaning. The results of such research were seen as difficult to apply in the context of human experience. Phenomenology, in contrast, seeks to understand and describe human experience (Leininger, 1985; Swanson-Kauffman and Schonwald, 1988). This is achieved by defining the reality of a situation, listening to individuals and their views, in their natural setting.

Phenomenology is a qualitative research method which generates knowledge that has value for people involved with people, as in nursing. Oiler (1982) and Leininger (1985) both advocate its use in nursing as they believe it conforms to the values of nursing. In my study the meaning of caring in the intensive care unit was clarified. The experience of caring can arise from the carer (the nurses), and those being cared for (the patient). The reality of caring for those participating is defined by listening to individuals and their views, expressed in their natural setting. This generates, through a process of rigorous analysis, a description of caring derived from individuals' personal knowledge gained through experience.

The phenomenological method uses an inductive descriptive approach to generate a model of experience, originating from the data obtained. This requires the experiencing person to speak about the phenomenon under study (Van Kaam, 1966). The outcome of phenomenological enquiry is reliant on the researcher's ability to engage in the participant's reality, 'as if' that reality were the researcher's own (Swanson-Kauffman and Schonwald, 1988). This requries the researcher 'to hear' what the experiencing person is saying.

Data collection

In light of the previous discussion the principal method of data collection used was unstructured interviews, I had hoped, of patients and nurses. Although this provided second-hand accounts of others' experiences, reconstructions of experience are filtered by perception, the richness and description of experiences from individuals' perspectives provides insights into the significance given to thoughts, feelings and actions related to that experience (Bogdan and Taylor, 1984). To complement further the data collected I chose to be an 'observer as participant', moving freely within the setting, with minimal participation in the work role. This helped to contextualize the interviews and develop a rapport with the staff, enabling me to identify with their everyday work world. 'Hearing' may be dependent upon comprehending the natural setting. Burgess (1984) suggests that familiarity with the setting may lead to oversimplification and prior judgements to be made. He argues that being an outsider, not known to the setting, gives the researcher scope to stand back, whereas Field and Morse (1985) suggest that being an insider, known to the setting, provides a better position to elicit meaning. The natural interactions arising from being an insider, promote a rapport with the participants, enabling them readily to share their experiences. In my study the intensive care unit involved was not the one in which my research question arose, however, it was an environment which was similar. The participants knew of me. The advantage of not being a stranger meant that my presence caused little disruption and much humour. The staff were accepting of me and they were able to relax and carry on with their work as normal, as this comment from my field notes illustrates:

> Although I feel awkward in my role as researcher, the staff appear comfortable and friendly when I am around, teasing me that I am a new James Bond . . . they continue doing the things they do as if I am one of them.

The participants

In my role as researcher I felt uncomfortable with those involved being known as informants. The tone I had wished to set for this study was one of sharing. Using the word participants in describing the sample I felt acknowledged this. The participants were those nurses who were primarily responsible for prescribing nursing care at the bedside. Although it was anticipated that those only at salary grades E and F would be interviewed, after informal discussion with the staff I decided to include also those staff at salary grade D. Nine of 22 eligible nurses volunteered to participate, all were registered general nurses, working as staff nurses, their length of experience in intensive care ranged from two months to 31 years. Their ages were between 22 and 50. Eight participants were female and one was male. While I had hoped to interview patients who had experienced mechanical ventilation in intensive care, the four potential participants had no recall of being in the intensive care unit. The intensive care unit contained five beds, was one of a purpose-built design and located in a district general hospital.

Triangulation

The concept of triangulation originates from the world of navigation and military strategy. Its purpose is to establish where your location is. It is a procedure that utilizes geometry by taking multiple reference points to locate an unknown position accurately (Mitchell, 1986). In research, triangulation may be defined as combining methods in a study which considers an unknown phenomenon. This may involve simple or complex processes dependent upon the level of triangulation the research design indicates. Mitchell (1986) describes a triangulated study as a combination of different theoretical perspectives, different data sources, different investigators, or different methods within a single study. Measurement from several vantage points supports comparison, allowing the phenomenon to be identified, the purpose of which is to promote the credibility of the study in terms of increasing reliability and validity, thus overcoming the deficiencies and biases that stem from any single research method. The aim of triangulation is to achieve results from which the information that is obtained reflects the phenomenon being studied rather than reflecting the method being used to measure the phenomenon (Mitchell, 1986; Duffy, 1987; Banik, 1993). The findings of the study are not method-bound and reflect the true nature of the phenomenon.

Triangulation may be seen as an attempt to enhance/compensate for the merits and limitations of both quantitative and qualitative research methods. Phenomena of interest to nursing initially have been studied using research methodologies arising from the quantitative domain of scientific enquiry. This approach emphasizes the search for facts and causes of human behaviour through objective, observable and quantifiable data. Knowledge is universal, arising from one reality which exists and can be measured using our senses; it is 'there to be found'. Finding the facts, however, involves creating an experiment or research tool to establish what the facts are. The situation is controlled or manipulated in an attempt to establish cause and effect, but from the perspective of the researcher. This reductionist view has often been criticized for not considering the meaning and context of the situation that may strongly influence human behaviour. Yet as an emerging academic discipline nursing, wishing to be accepted and respected in the scientific community, was strongly influenced by this dominant view of science. The prevailing climate encouraged this view of science to be utilized.

Duffy (1987) highlights the disenchantment nurse researchers have felt when trying to understand people and their health care needs and problems when using quantitative research methods. The values within this dominant paradigm of research conflict with the values held in nursing; that a person cannot be reduced to component parts; that the meaning and the context of their situation will influence their actions and ultimately their health. This caused a shift to utilizing qualitative research methods which study the world from the perspective of the subjects. This approach emphasizes the subjective view of the world. Multiple realities co-exist arising from our perceptions of the situation, and these research methods consider the 'as I see it' perspective. Knowledge is personal and arises from values, meanings, beliefs, thoughts, feelings, and general characteristics pertaining to a phenomenon of interest. No attempt to control or manipulate the events of the situation is made. Triangulation may be used as an attempt to marry the differences between these two fundamentally different research paradigms, to gain an accurate objective and subjective view of a phenomenon in question.

Nursing's fascination with triangulation has emerged recently, arising from the scientific necessity fully to understand phenomena of concern to nursing (Sohier, 1988). Yet Duffy (1987) suggests that this fascination may be a position of appeasement to the purist perspectives held within each of the research domains described above. Verification and discovery are both processes which can be used to define phenomenon and have value for nursing (Banik, 1993). Combining these processes through the use of triangulation may provide a more complete picture of the phenomenon under question.

Triangulation may strengthen a research study design. Denzin (1989) suggests that no single method in research fully examines a phenomenon, because each differing method reveals a different aspect of reality, therefore multiple methods should be employed to research a phenomenon. The integration and mixing of research methods and theoretical perspectives counterbalances the weaknesses of one method with the strengths of the other(s) used. Mitchell (1986) asserts that such integration of method promotes the understanding of complex phenomena, that triangulation is a suitable strategy to use in nursing research. Triangulation is an ideal that promotes creativity in research design by the mixing and matching of research methods to produce new, deeper understandings of the phenomenon of concern (Patton, 1990). Denzin (1989) identifies four types of triangulation, data, investigator, theory and methodological, that can be used in the research process (see Figure 8.1).

Data triangulation is the use of a variety sources of data within one study. The data collected are dissimilar but with a common focus and sources of data may be across individuals, different times of day and different settings, for example, when considering caring, talking to patients and nurses, observation of nurse–patient interactions during different shifts and completing the research in different ward/departments. The data obtained are rich and diverse, once examined, differences and similarities provide greater understanding of the dimensions of the phenomenon across people, places and time.

Investigator triangulation is the use of several investigators with different expertise. The mixture of knowledge and experience this provides within a study when working with the raw data reduces the potential bias that may occur in a single investigator study. The multiple interpretations of the data produce a high degree of corroboration, increasing the reliability of the study (Banik, 1993) and Duffy (1987) noted that this method of triangulation reduces premature closing about the meaning of a phenomenon. A single investigator may become tired and exhausted with the data collected before the collection processes have become saturated, producing no new information in relation to the phenomenon under examination. These gains are said to outweigh the difficulties in obtaining inter-investigator reliability (Banik, 1993).

Theory triangulation is the use of multiple perspectives to analyse and interpret a single set of data. For example, when considering the content of interviews about caring, using Leininger's (1985) theory of transcultural care and Watson's (1979) theory of caring to analyse the data may provide

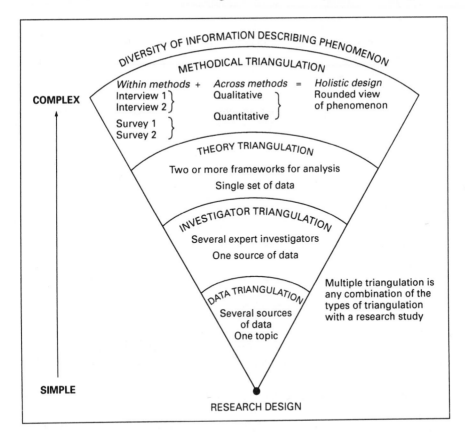

Figure 8.1   Types of triangulation

common areas of caring which satisfy both cultural and interpersonal dimensions of the phenomenon. This increases the significance and practical use of the results of the study.

Finally, methodological triangulation is the use of multiple methods to study a single phenomenon and could be either 'within methods', 'across methods' or 'holisitc design', each increasing the complexity of triangulation within the study design. Within methods triangulation is the use of similar techniques within one research domain to collect data; this aids comparison of the information collected. The mixing of qualitative and quantitative methods would achieve across methods triangulation. Participant observation or interview content could be analysed against the content of a structured questionnaire. Holistic design incorporates within methods triangulation, both qualitative and quantitative, then across method triangulation of the results obtained from within methods triangulation is achieved (see Figure 8.2). Jick (1983) argues that the high degree of complexity of this approach increases the validity of the findings,

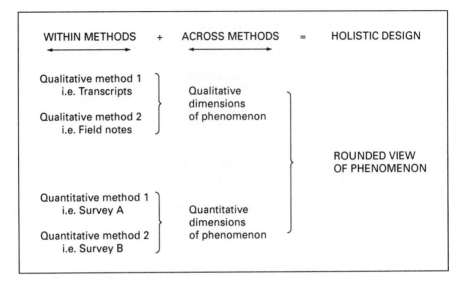

Figure 8.2 Methodological triangulation

providing confidence in the data ascertained being fully representative of the phenomenon being considered due to convergence of the data achieved by the use of multiple triangulation.

Triangulation was a concept introduced to me during the research methods course within my degree studies. In essence I wished to cross-check the data I obtained from different qualitative methods used for data collection. Within the research process this would occur usually after the data collection phase, during data analysis. In terms of my own study the idea appeared simple and I hoped triangulation would affirm the validity of my research study's findings. Kimchi *et al.* (1991) state that the goal of triangulation is to circumvent the personal bias and deficiencies intrinsic to a single-investigator study. Given the nature of the phenomenon I was considering I wanted to be sure the results reflected the views held by the participants, not the views held by myself, the researcher. In my study I had planned to complete three sources of data collection: interviewing the nurses; interviewing the patients and observation of the setting. This would comply with Denzin's (1989) description of within-methods triangulation, when multiple methods of data collection are used to view the same phenomenon.

At the level of analysis only two sources of data were available to me: the transcripts from the interviews I had completed with the nurses and my fieldnotes from my periods of observation. During the process of analysis I realized that I had two different types of data informing me of different facets of caring: an insider's perspective of caring and an outsider's perspective of caring. These seemed to me two different facets of the phenomenon which could not be compared. The following are illustrations taken from similar incidents. The first taken from a transcript offers an insider's perspective of caring:

> You can tell when a patient's distressed, you can see it, take Sam when he needs to cough, you can hear the secretions on his chest, but you know if you suck him out he'll get more distressed and go red in the face because the ET tube is irritating his throat, so you explain to him that if you clear his chest he will feel more comfortable, you have to be quick, get the agony over with, so you talk him through it whilst you're doing it, even though he can't respond . . . you settle him down, make sure everything's connected, stay with him, holding his hand, soothing him until he calms.

The second taken from the fieldnotes offers an outsider's perspective:

> The ventilator alarmed. Jo went over, looked at the ventilator settings, then turned the alarm off, and moved behind the head of the bed. Jo checked her support equipment. Glove in hand she armed herself with a suction catheter, she stood at the head of the bed and carried out the procedure of endotracheal suction, efficiently and effectively. She reconnected the ventilator circuit and reset the alarm, then carried out oropharyngeal suction, after the suction catheter was in and out, and the procedure almost done, Jo said 'I'm just going to clear your mouth'. Once finished Jo cleared away the used equipment and returned to her chart. She appeared intent on completing the task.

Triangulation it seemed was not appropriate as the two accounts bore no resemblance to each other. I had different accounts of experience (Reason and Rowan, 1981). Phenomenology is a description of being in the world from the conscious position of those experiencing it. To triangulate knowledge obtained from experience would require data from first-person descriptions. But with observation I am not sharing that experience, I was just 'seeing' it from my perspective as researcher. I didn't have that first-person experience to use as a source of data. Phenomenology is the use of subjective and first-person experience as a source of knowledge, sharing that 'being in the world'. The first-person account shared with me the participant's experience. To achieve within-method triangulation of my data, I would need to experience caring as a nurse in that setting, obtaining first-person knowledge by participating in managing patient care. This was reflected and confirmed in my fieldnotes of one evening when I became involved in patient care:

> 'Janet, I can hear that you want to cough', Janet is deeply sedated and cannot respond. I move around the back of the bed 'Janet I know you can't see me. I'm going to be as quick as I can; this may feel quite strange.' I get my equipment ready, now ready to start, I place a hand gently on the forehead of the patient, using alternate hands I gently stroke Janet's forehead, I turn her head from side to side, checking the tape . . . not touching the distant end of the suction catheter I insert it into the endotracheal tube; the noise is like sucking hard on a straw but the liquid won't come up easily. My left hand is always in

contact with the patient's face and the right hand removing the catheter. I repeat the whole process, the tube is clear, less than a minute later Janet is connected to the ventilator again, I stay holding her hand until her vital signs settle.

My experience echoed that offered as the first example, but again was different from the observations made in my fieldnotes. The outsider view may not be the same phenomenon. Although triangulation was operationally correct according to Denzin (1989), my research design highlighted that I may not be viewing the same phenomenon if I were to remain true to the methodology chosen for my study. What I saw and what I felt were distinctly different, therefore the observation data I had collected in my fieldnotes had to be abandoned in respect of using them in the data analysis for the purposes of triangulation. Within phenomenology my choice of observer-as-participant highlighted the differences between first- and third-person knowledge. My research design highlighted the need for first-person experience to be obtained if triangulation were to be achieved. However, the opportunity to observe was not without value, as through this method I was able to become familiar with the intensive care unit and staff. Observation offered contextual information to the study in relation to the data obtained, allowing me to set the scene and understand the experience of caring from the perspective of others.

Triangulation can be a powerful solution to the problem of relying on any single data source or method within a research study, but certain principles must guide its use. The research question needs to be focused, providing a clear direction for the research design. The methods used should be complementary, providing balance for the inherent strengths and weaknesses in the methods chosen. The methods should be relevant to the nature of the phenomenon under study and evaluation of the research process should be continuous, the researcher being in touch with the data obtained and the theory being used within the study. Triangulation requires thorough planning and meticuluous attention to detail. In analysing my own experience in trying to use triangulation, while I had chosen a relatively simple approach to test I had not accounted for the discrepancies between the theoretical underpinning of my study and the process of triangulation. The mixing of qualitative data collection methods against the internal consistency and logic of phenomenology caused a dilemma, one mitigated against the other, causing for me a methodological controversy. I had to decide which I would pursue, triangulation or phenomenology. Reviewing the purpose of the study and considering the moral obligations I felt towards matching a methodology that was pertinent to the nature of the phenomenon, the research question and the values that had strongly influenced my original decision in using phenomenology I erred on the side of being a purist to the methodology I had chosen. Banik (1993) argues that a researcher needs to be open to more than one way of looking at things, but in this instance to have such breadth of vision would compromise the research design, invalidating the contributions of the participants. I decided to respect the participants' views and value the meanings given to me in relation to the concept of caring, honouring the philosophical stance held within phenomenology. This meant 'losing' data, that were available to me in the fieldnotes I had taken. This source of data could not be used in the data analysis of the study.

I had set out at the start of my study to establish the meaning of caring, what I heard and what I saw were two different representations of reality, the difference between words and actions: the insider perspective conflicting with the outsider perspective. If I had chosen to use ethnography or grounded theory as the methodology to underpin my research study, then the issue of mixing at the analysis level would not have caused such conflict. I chose to be pure to the method for the philosophical reasons discussed earlier. With hindsight I realize now that the dilemma posed to me originated from a fundamental clash of the beliefs within the two methods, triangulation and phenomenology, chosen. Duffy's (1987) idea that triangulation has arisen in response to the dominant view of science to objectify qualitative studies, decries the value of seeking out and understanding a person's subjective experience. Triangulation may encourage the researcher to focus on 'parts' rather than the 'whole' in the rigour of cross-checking and analysing the data. There were practical gains in being a purist to the method of phenomenology; it reduced the amount of data I had to analyse in a short time frame. While the idea of triangulation in this instance was sound, I was an inexperienced researcher who had not acknowledged the potential complexity triangulation brings to any study. I had wanted the world to know that I had used strategies to reduce bias and increase the validity of the findings, yet in being true to the values implicit in using phenomenology this was not necessary. I had a description of the meaning of caring from first-person experience, which could only be triangulated by others' first-hand experience, namely the patients or other nurses. The advantage of using triangulation lies in the increased credibility the findings have for exploring a phenomenon, yet the potential complexity of the processes involved and the expense this may have in time, monies and tools used are disadvantages to be considered carefully in the planning stage of any research project.

Data analysis

Rigour within phenomenology arises in capturing adequately, succinctly and creatively the lived experience of caring for those involved. It became apparent to me that data analysis was an act of interpretation by the researcher which represents the participants' description of caring. The data inductively obtained from the interviews became the focus of analysis. Structured reflections, through phenomenological reduction, a process of reducing the data obtained from the nine participants to one description of caring in this study, provides an opportunity to examine caring as it arises from the meanings given to it as it is experienced rather than considering caring from a conceptual basis. This facilitates an understanding of caring and the discovery of beliefs, attitudes and intuitions held by the participants about caring.

During the reductive process it was important to remain faithful to the words and meanings as described by the participants themselves. To help achieve this I used a process of phenomenological reduction outlined by Colaizzi (1978) to complete my data analysis, which is described below:

- The transcripts are read individually to gain a sense of the whole.
- Significant statements and phrases pertaining to the phenomenon under study are extracted from each transcript.
- Meanings are formulated from the significant statements, but not in isolation of the original transcripts.
- Themes and theme clusters are developed, referring to the original transcripts in order to validate them and note discrepancies.
- A description of the phenomenon from the integration of the results obtained is provided.
- The essential structure of the phenomenon is derived.
- Validation is sought from the participants to compare the descriptive results with their experience.

Analysing the data was a lengthy process, as each transcript was considered many times. To take the narrative of thousands of words down to one description of caring which would be an accurate representation of the stories given to me about caring seemed an impossible task. I read the verbatim transcripts and listened to the tape recordings simultaneously to acquire a sense of the whole interview and to clarify the meanings obtained from the words of each participant. Once the significant statements were extracted from each transcript, accuracy of the significant statements was checked by re-reading the original transcripts. Swanson-Kauffman and Schonwald (1988) highlighted that intuiting the meanings within these statements requires time for consideration and reflection. Formulating meanings moves the participants' narrative to precised statements reflecting their meanings; for me this was an intensive process which took many hours and much angst as I wondered if I had retained the essence of the meanings given to me. I generated 89 'formulated meanings' from the 619 significant statements taken from the transcripts earlier in my analysis. Groupings began to emerge, tentative themes and theme cluster names originated from the participants' own words and meanings given to me, continuing the process of reduction (see Figure 8.3).

Constant throughout the process was the cross-checking back and forth between each stage to ensure that the data had only been reduced and not altered. The rigour implicit within this process promoted the internal

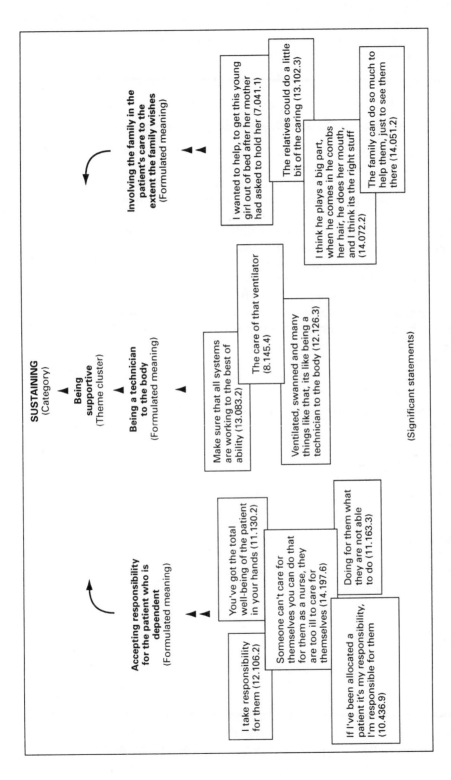

SUSTAINING
(Category)

Being supportive
(Theme cluster)

Accepting responsibility for the patient who is dependent
(Formulated meaning)

Being a technician to the body
(Formulated meaning)

Involving the family in the patient's care to the extent the family wishes
(Formulated meaning)

I take responsibility for them (12.106.2)

You've got the total well-being of the patient in your hands (11.130.2)

Someone can't care for themselves you can do that for them as a nurse, they are too ill to care for themselves (14.197.6)

If I've been allocated a patient it's my responsibility, I'm responsible for them (10.436.9)

Doing for them what they are not able to do (11.163.3)

Make sure that all systems are working to the best of ability (13.083.2)

The care of that ventilator (8.145.4)

Ventilated, swanned and many things like that, its like being a technician to the body (12.126.3)

I wanted to help, to get this young girl out of bed after her mother had asked to hold her (7.041.1)

The relatives could do a little bit of the caring (13.102.3)

I think he plays a big part, when he comes in he combs her hair, he does her mouth, and I think its the right stuff (14.072.2)

The family can do so much to help them, just to see them there (14.051.2)

(Significant statements)

Figure 8.3 An example of developing categories from significant statements

validity of the study. Krefting (1991) highlighted that for qualitative research methods validity is viewed from the perspective of trustworthiness of the propositons made; that the final description truly represented the meanings of caring given to me. Staying true to the data is important to ensure that no additional constructs alter the data. Through the process of interpretation the researcher may inadvertently add their own views and meanings to the analysis. Analysing the data continued the process of bracketing (Oiler, 1982) for me as it became evident that in reducing the data down to theme clusters I had pieces that didn't fit! I had written each 'formulated meaning' on a catalogue card and began sorting them into categories, only to find that I had seven cards which would not fit into the categories identified. No matter how I sorted the cards, these seven would not fit, until I realized that I had filtered the data through predetermined categories I had read about in the literature, loosely named as caring, not caring and factors that hindered caring. Abandoning these categories because they had not originated from the participants' meanings meant I started my analysis from the beginning again. I felt I had to start again to establish where these additional constructs had crept into the description I was trying to elicit and to ensure that I had been true to the data from the beginning; the findings of this second more accurate analysis can be found in Table 8.1.

The only way I would finally know that the representation of caring I had generated had been true to the data would be when the participants read the description and told me so, fulfilling Bronfenbrenner's (1976) idea that feedback from the participants provides a source of feedback that promotes the internal validity of a study utilizing phenomenological enquiry. Sandelowski (1986) suggests that a qualitative study is credible when it presents such accurate descriptions or interpretation of human experience that people who also share that experience would immediately recognize the descriptions. The nine participants all provided feedback and agreed that the exhaustive description of caring presented below represented the experience and the meanings they gave to that experience. One comment by a participant summed it up by saying: 'Yep, that's it . . . in a nut-shell!' At the time relief flooded through me that I had been true to the data given to me; now I would say 'What a nut-shell!'

Others' views

For the nurses within this study caring involved being at the bedside with the patient, taking on responsibility for the totally dependent person. Despite the gravity of the situation, caring involved making the effort to address the individual's needs, and being the patient's spokesperson within the team. The practical activity of caring includes giving nursing care and technical support, both are constant and essential to the process of

Table 8.1 Descriptive components of the phenomenon of caring

Category	Theme cluster	Themes (formulated meanings)
Being involved	Being there	Putting the patient first before the routine
		Sharing feelings and emotion with the patient and the family
		Making time to be with the patient
		Letting them (the relative) talk
		Making an effort to communicate with patients whether conscious or unconscious
		The physical presence of the nurse
		Being available to the patient
		Being recognized by the patient
	Being close	You make meaning with, being involved with the patient
		Using touch affectionately to display warmth and tenderness
		Giving the patient loving affection
		Being a friend
		Doing the 'little things'
		Being honest
		Creating the a picture of who they are
		Being remembered by the patient and family
	Respecting the person	Recognizing each patient as a person with individual needs
		Being honest
		Value the trust given
		Relating to the person
		Acknowledging the patient's presence
		Returning the responsibility to the patient, when they are able to take it, within the boundaries of their illness
	Feeling for	Having hope
		Putting self in the patient's position to try and ascertain how the patient is feeling and wants to be cared for
		Caring is acknowledging death as a part of life and feeling for the loss of that person
	Involving family	Caring for the family is as important as caring for the patient
		Using feedback from relatives to evaluate care
		Explaining every aspect of care to the patient and the family
		Acknowledging and alleviating the patient's and the family's fear from being in intensive care
		Letting the family stay
		Involving the family in the patient's care to the extent the family wishes

Table 8.1 continued

Category	Theme cluster	Themes (formulated meanings)
Sustaining	Being supportive	Accepting responsibility for the patient who is dependent
		Working closely with nursing colleagues and other disciplines
		Knowing about the patient's condition, care and possible outcomes
		Letting the patient rest
		Being a technician to the body
		Doing your best for the patient
		Attending to the basic needs of the patient
		Looking after your staff
		Carrying out physical tasks and duties
		Being the patient's advocate so that the patient's needs are apparent to all concerned
		Letting the family stay
		Involving the family in the patient's care to the extent the family wishes
		Supporting colleagues
		Assessing the patient's condition accurately, anticipating and being able to act on that information
		Giving the patient what they want or need
		Making the patient comfortable
		Acknowledging and alleviating the patient's and the family's fear from being in intensive care
		Explaining every aspect of care to the patient and the family
	Having experience	Having experience of nursing
		Caring qualities of parents
		The nurse having been a patient admitted to hospital
		Caring as a way of life
		Inexperience reduces confidence and affects ability to care
		Inherent ability and personal attributes of nurse influences caring
	Gaining expertise	Taking on an extra developmental role
		Variety of work challenging
		Asking questions, sharing and contributing ideas enhances learning
		Gaining knowledge through attendance on study days and courses
		Having in-house teaching sessions and supervision
		Role modelling of caring attributes and skills
		Mentoring students
		Too many roles depletes the energy available for caring
		Lack of knowledge detracts from nurse's ability to care

Table 8.1   continued

Category	Theme cluster	Themes (formulated meanings)
	Feelings about work	Being valued by the team increases the nurse's sense of self-worth
		Accomplishment gives satisfaction
		Enjoyment in life away from work enhances caring
		Being able to isolate emotions in difficult situations helps the nurse when caring
		Having an 'off day'
		Negative attitudes arising from colleagues causes demoralization
	Resources	Having time to care
		Having routines
		Appropriate staffing establishment
		Being well equipped
		Having one patient to care for
Being frustrated	Rigors	Relatives becoming a nuisance
		Aggressive patients and relatives
		Agitated, unsettled patients
		Patients not able to communicate
	Constraints	Lack of facilities for relatives
		Interruptions
		The routine taking precedence
		Writing care-plans
		Lack of organization
		Not having enough time
		Inappropriate staffing levels
		Having more than one patient to care for
		Lack of autonomy
	Difficulties within team	Lack of leadership
		Poor communication amongst team
		Others not acknowledging patient as a person
		Not getting constructive feedback on performance
		Nurses' needs paramount to patients' needs
		Lack of understanding and support from medical team
		Negative attitudes arising from colleagues causes demoralization

caring. Emotional caring, having feelings for the patient, is dependent upon the relationships formed with the patient and/or the family. When personally involved, physical care is given with emotional warmth. Caring for the family is a component of caring for the patient, and is achieved by supporting and involving the family in caring.

The nurse brings inherent abilities and attitudes to the process of caring;

these arise from life experience and professional learning. To continue to care, without personal cost to the nurse, professional growth, resources and support from colleagues are required. Caring is enhanced by feeling good, but energies available for caring are reduced when frustrations are experienced at work. In these situations the nurse continues to give physical caring, but the level of emotional caring is reduced. The nurse feeling cared for has the motivation to care for others.

This chapter illustrates the complexity of triangulation. While I understood the idea and had planned to use triangulation in a simple form, experiences of doing research highlighted the difficulties in applying the concept to practice. My study design may have been ambitious to begin with; coupled with my innocence of the research process in action, I had learnt that not all ideas can be carried through. Situations and learning present choices in the research process and each decision made has a weight to it, what may be gained and what may be lost. For me, the advantages of being a 'purist' outweighed the advantages of 'mixing' methods to explore the phenomenon of caring. This decision was based on the values inherent within the methodology I had chosen to use, enabling me to listen to the thoughts, feelings and actions surrounding caring by those nurses involved in caring, keeping in mind the question I was asking. Protecting the potency of the nurses' perspective within this research study provided credibility of a difference sense to that associated with triangulation – accepting and representing their word accurately was enough within this research design. Utilizing a qualitative methodology allowed the research process, for me, to be dynamic and responsive to the issues and decisions involved when carrying out research. Triangulation is a method which has value for the research process if complementary to the underpinning methodology used within the research project's design.

All names used in this chapter are pseudonyms.

References

Banik B J (1993) Applying triangulation in nursing research. *Applied Nursing Research* 6 (1), 47–52.

Bronfenbrenner U (1976) The experimental ecology of education. *Teachers' College Record* 78 (2), 157–78.

Burgess R G (1984) *In the Field: An Introduction to Field Research.* Allen & Unwin, London.

Colaizzi P G (1978) Psychological research as the phenomenologist views it. In Valle R S and King M (Eds) *Existential Phenomenological Alternatives for Psychology.* Oxford University Press, Oxford, pp. 48–71.

Denzin N K (1989) *The Research Act,* 3rd edn. McGraw-Hill, New York.

Drew N (1989) The interviewer's experience as data in phenomenological research. *Western Journal of Nursing Research* 11 (4), 431–9.

Duffy M E (1987) Methodological triangulation: a vehicle for merging quantitative and qualitative research methods. *Image: Journal of Nursing Scholarship* 19 (3), 130–3.

Field P A and Morse J M (1985) *Nursing Research. The Application of Qualitative Approaches.* Chapman & Hall, London.

Jick T (1983) Mixing qualitative and quantitative methods: triangulation in action. In J Van Maanen (Ed.) *Qualitative Methodology.* Sage, Newbury Park, CA, pp. 135–48.

Kimchi J, Polivka B, and Stevenson J S (1991) Triangulation: operational definitions. *Nursing Research* 40 (6), 364–6.

Krefting L (1991) Rigor in qualitative research. The assessment of trustworthiness. *American Journal of Occupational Therapy* 45 (3), 214–22.

Leininger M M (Ed.) (1985) *Qualitative Research Methods in Nursing.* Grune & Stratton, Orlando, FL.

Melia K M (1982) 'Tell it as it is' – qualitative methodology and nursing research: understanding the student nurse's world. *Journal of Advanced Nursing* 7 (4), 327–35.

Mitchell E S (1986) Multiple triangulation: a methodology for nursing science. *Advances in Nursing Science* 8 (3), 18–26.

Moccia P (1988) A critique of compromise: beyond the methods debate. *Advances in Nursing Science* 10 (4), 1–9.

Oiler C (1982) The phenomenological approach in nursing research. *Nursing Research* 31 (3), 178–81.

Omery A (1983) Phenomenology: a method for nursing research. *Advances in Nursing Science* 5 (2), 49–63.

Patton M Q (1990) *Qualitative Evaluation and Research Methods,* 2nd edn. Sage, Newbury Park, CA.

Reason P and Rowan J (Eds) (1981) *Human Inquiry. A Sourcebook of New Paradigm Research.* John Wiley, Chichester.

Sandelowski M (1986) The problem of rigor in qualitative research. *Advances in Nursing Science* 8 (3), 27–37.

Sohier R (1988) Multiple triangulation and contemporary nursing research. *Western Journal of Nursing Research* 10 (6), 732–42.

Spiegelberg H (1976) *The Phenomenological Movement,* Vol. 2. Martinus Nijhoff, The Hague.

Swanson-Kauffman K and Schonwald E (1988) Phenomenology. In Sarter B (Ed.), *Paths to Knowledge: Innovative Research Methods for Nursing.* National League for Nursing, New York, pp. 97–105.

Taylor S J and Bogdan, R (1984) *Introduction to Qualitative Research Methods: The Search for Meanings,* 2nd edn. John Wiley, New York.

Van Kaam A (1966) *Existential Foundations of Psychology.* Image Books, New York.

Watson J (1979) *Nursing: The Philosophy and Science of Caring.* Little Brown and Co., Boston, MA.

9

Relationships – who needs them?
A study of teachers' learning styles
and teaching strategies

Pat Le Rolland

The mention of quantitative research, hypothesis and correlation techniques are likely to switch many an avid student of research off. However, this chapter:

- *contrasts approaches to the survey method in Chapter 7;*
- *explores questionnaire design and offers some useful suggestions;*
- *explains correlation techniques and applies them to the findings;*
- *the conclusion contains positive suggestions on the way forward for the novice and experienced researcher.*

Introduction

The research underpinning this chapter explores what the relationship is between the teaching strategies that teachers use in classroom settings and their personal learning styles in one Faculty. This chapter discusses quantitative research methods by the exploration of a study which used correlation techniques on data gained from a survey. The aim is to highlight some of the experiences of a teacher as a researcher in relation to quantitative analysis; the study itself is not related in detail but some of the results are shown in order to inform the discussion and hopefully make the work more meaningful for the reader. There are many forms of quantitative research and this work does not claim to be comprehensive. What I do hope is that it helps readers to avoid some of the pitfalls and to consider the fact that quantitative research still has an important role in nursing and nursing education.

The first part of the chapter gives a concise overview of the research and goes on to discuss the process of deciding upon the research question. There is a brief examination of learning styles, and how teaching strategies were operationalized in the study.

The issue of research design and methodology is then analysed. As questionnaires were the main data collection tool they are discussed in more detail. There is specific examination of Honey and Mumford's learning style questionnaire (1992) revised in 1986, with some thoughts on the accompanying letters when using postal questionnaires. The next part of the chapter discusses the use of self-designed questionnaires and particularly the one used in the study to ascertain the teaching strategies used by the respondents.

The pilot process and results are reviewed, followed by a crucial aspect of the study which was to designate teaching strategies to learning styles. There will then be a scrutiny of the results leading to some recommendations.

In conclusion the key aspects of the study will be drawn together and some issues related to learning styles, questionnaires and quantitative research put forward for consideration. Suggestions for helpful texts will be included, and the context of future research in nursing and nursing education highlighted.

Overview

The aim of this study was to ascertain what the relationship is between the teaching strategies that teachers use in the classroom setting, and their personal learning styles in one Faculty (formerly a College of Health Care Studies). A review of the literature revealed a need for further study into why teachers choose certain teaching strategies to inform the debate about learning style preferences and how teaching styles and learning orientations could be related.

The study used correlation techniques on data gained by a survey of the nurse teachers. Assessment of teachers' learning styles was undertaken using a learning style questionnaire (Honey and Mumford, 1992) and teaching strategies were self-reported for a 10-day period using an author-designed questionnaire. The strategies were classified into four categories of activities based on the association with a particular learning style.

Data analysis revealed that the Faculty staff were evenly distributed for three of the four learning styles (reflector, theorist and pragmatist) in comparison with occupational norms, but only a fifth of the teachers had an activist learning style preference. A minority of the teachers showed moderate or strong preferences in all four styles, i.e. that they could be said to be all-rounders, being adaptable and benefiting from new learning experiences. A wide range of all defined teaching strategies was reported, with student-centred activities being most frequently used; however, some of the teachers did not use any teaching strategies linked with certain learning styles.

No significant correlation was found and the results of the study indicated that teachers' learning styles did not influence their choice of strategy.

It was recommended that further study should examine other factors that affect the teaching/learning situation and that the style and skill with which a teacher approaches any teaching method are crucial to successful learning.

The research question

Arriving at a conclusion as to what the study was really and fully about was one of the hardest aspects of the research process. An initial interest in learning styles grew from reading and from the work setting where students had the opportunity to explore their own learning styles in order to facilitate efficient learning and studying. The examination of learning styles of students had generated a wide range of data in general education, occupational training and to a lesser extent in nursing education. Kolb (1984) and Honey and Mumford (1992) embed their work in the four-stage experiential learning cycle (see Figure 9.1) and identify learning orientations or preferences. It is argued that people learn more effectively if their learning style preferences are acknowledged by themselves and their teachers (Honey and Mumford, 1992), although there has been debate as to whether teachers should match or mismatch their teaching approaches (Dunn and Dunn, 1979; Partridge, 1983; McMillan and Dwyer, 1990). Partridge (1983) outlines some potential matches ranging from compensatory (trying to circumvent student 'deficiencies') to challenge (deliberate mismatch of the teaching approach in order to encourage expansion of the student's learning style repertoire).

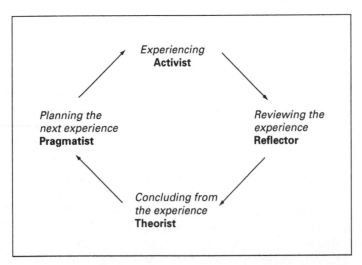

Figure 9.1   Honey and Mumford's four-stage experiential learning cycle

Further reading revealed two main presumptions: first, that identification and utilization of students' learning styles was seen as a fundamental need, without any reference to the teacher's own learning styles, and secondly that teachers will alter their teaching strategies according to the students' needs and in a skilful and responsive manner.

From the writer's experience, particularly with the much larger student cohorts being taught in lecture theatres, the idea of adapting one's teaching to students' learning styles is adhered to more in spirit rather than in reality. With developments such as open and distance learning teachers are likely to require staff development programmes that increase their range of teaching approaches. As cost effectiveness is a key issue within health care and education systems the time and money used to update teachers could be more effective if the same concern was shown about the learning styles of teachers as it is for the students!

A note of caution is needed at this point – as I was clarifying what I wished to investigate, the literature, in my novice opinion, was revealing an area of valid research yet through experience I would advise that one considers why this particular aspect of research has not been undertaken. One reason could be that it is not possible to identify the 'answer'.

The final stage of deciding on the hypothesis was to be explicit about the terms under investigation, clear operational definitions being vital for research as a communication process (Tuckman, 1988). As I had decided to use Honey and Mumford's (1992) learning style questionnaire their definition of learning styles was used: 'The term learning styles is used as a description of the attitudes and behaviours which determine an individual's preferred way of learning' (Honey and Mumford, 1992, p. 1). This was a useful as well as convenient choice as it makes it clear that students can learn in a variety of ways but that some are easier than others, it acknowledges that a learning style preference is not static and that learning is affective in nature.

The activities that a teacher undertakes within the classroom have been described as teaching styles, teaching methods and teaching strategies. On examination, teaching methods could mean a range of aspects from the visual aids used to the overall educational philosophy underpinning practice, an ambiguity highlighted by Bligh (1971). Teaching styles had been studied as a cognitive trait (Joyce and Hudson, 1968), as an influence on students' approach to studying (Lapeyre, 1992) and had been used interchangeably with teaching strategies (e.g. Laschinger *et al.*, 1986).

Finally I defined a teaching strategy as:

A particular method of teaching within an overall teaching/learning experience, i.e. the actual behaviours initiated and planned for by the teacher.

Having become clearer about what I wished to investigate and that the learning style questionnaire produced numerical data, then correlation research within a survey approach seemed to be the way to test my hypothesis: that if there was a strong or low preference shown in a particular learning style then a correlation would reveal a high or low use of teaching strategies related to that learning style.

Research design and methodology

The design of the research was determined by the aim, the characteristics of the data to be examined and the practical constraints under which the data collection occurred.

Correlation research involves collecting data and finding if there is a relationship between them; a positive relationship is where a higher score in one set of data leads to a higher score in the other (Anderson, 1990). The Pearson product-moment correlation can be used for linear relationships and the coefficient (r) ranges from minus one to plus one with nought being no relationship between the two variables (Anderson, 1990). In this study the learning style was considered to be the independent variable and the teaching strategies the dependent variable. Correlation research is said to be a useful technique when exploring new issues when there are a large number of variables (Cohen and Manion, 1989; Anderson, 1990). The other advantages are that it can use data gained in a naturalist setting and that it does not require large samples (Cohen and Manion, 1989).

Disadvantages include the fact that a direct relationship is not proven even if a strongly positive correlation is shown, and therefore cause and effect are not established. Equally, enabling teachers to become more aware of their learning styles and to broaden their repertoire may not necessarily lead to a broader repertoire of teaching strategies. A final note of caution is that even if a statistically significant relationship is found, how significant is it to the overall teaching/learning environment?

As well as deciding upon what data will be gathered the research needs to communicate and justify what is considered but not included.

Questionnaires

Questionnaires as a research tool can be treated with insufficient care through familiarity. They can be postal questionnaires, group or self-administered or actual interview schedules, also they may contain checklists, rating or attitude scales (Oppenheim, 1992). It is the specification of the questionnaire that decides what it is measuring (Oppenheim, 1992).

Questionnaires are supposed to be free from interviewer bias (Macleod Clark and Hockey, 1979), but the design and use of the questions can be considered to contain researcher bias (Oppenheim, 1992). Well constructed questionnaires can be time and cost effective and produce reasonably valid data (Anderson, 1990), indeed in educational enquiry postal questionnaires can be considered the best form of survey, in comparison to interviews (Cohen and Manion, 1989). In order to be effective questionnaires must be attractive, clear and encourage maximum cooperation – simple to say but not to do. There is still debate as to the response rates in postal questionnaires; Oppenheim (1992) says that response rates can be low but Cohen and Manion (1989) consider this to be exaggerated. It is certainly true that a reminder must be planned for and considered an essential part of the research process.

Honey and Mumford's learning style questionnaire

There are 80 questions, 20 for each of the four learning styles which the respondent is asked to tick where they agree (or more than they disagree) with a statement, and cross if they disagree. The decision to use this questionnaire for the study was based on the fact that it is British, and therefore culturally more appropriate. It does not directly ask how the individual learns, which can be an advantage when teachers are the population under investigation, and it is said to be more user-friendly than the Kolb Learning Style Inventory (Honey and Mumford, 1992). It is said to have high reliability but with differences between learning styles, activists being most inconsistent (Honey and Mumford, 1992). Although face validity is considered to be high, technical validity has not been proven (Honey and Mumford, 1992). A key factor in deciding to use this questionnaire is that Honey and Mumford had norms for nurse teachers making analysis of the data more credible and that it has been used on a large population (n = 3500).

Prior to sending the questionnaire out to the nurse teachers (n = 74) I tried it out on myself and found that it only took about 10 minutes to complete, but another 10 to find out the scores and read the interpretation. Some questions were apparently repetitive and I realized that if one question was missed then it would make the use of that individual's data inappropriate. I also felt that the respondents would need to be offered the results as an incentive, but not on a free-for-all approach, or I would be incurring more cost and time in an activity not essential to the research process.

A flaw in the study lay in the fact that I did not pilot this questionnaire. This was not because I wished to change the tool but because when undertaking quantitative research the key point was to give oneself data to explore and 'play with'. By only piloting the other questionnaire I had to make up data in order to experience the actual correlation exercise for myself and consider the implications of the 'results'.

Accompanying letters

When deciding to use postal questionnaires the literature does not tend to give clear guidelines on what to put in the accompanying letter and yet I would argue that this aspect will improve the response rate and ensure the ethical code is followed. The letter needed to make it clear who I was, why I was doing this study, what I was asking the respondent to do, and to include enclosures such as the questionnaire itself, the return envelope and (in my research) a request for volunteers for the next stage of the study. This latter request also had to be user-friendly, and not expect the respondent to have to write an answer. Therefore it necessitated another document confirming on a yes/no basis whether he/she would participate in the teaching strategies exercise. It also had to confirm confidentiality, and that respondents could receive the personal results on the data of their learning styles. A further important point was that I intended to use the internal postal system, yet in order to maintain confidentiality the envelopes needed to be sealable, and this was an additional cost and time factor that I had underestimated. Personalizing the letters can help the response rate, and so I ensured the name of the respondents and my own name were handwritten. This can be done at the same time as coding the questionnaire.

When designing the first letter, I found it helpful to prepare the reminder letter at the same time. Tuckman (1988) recommends that if less than 80 per cent of the questionnaires are completed and returned then a follow-up should be attempted. A practical consideration is that one is trying to record the first respondents' data as well as sending out reminders, and the tone of the letter requires careful thought, it should be pleasant but not pleading, reminding respondents that this is the second request and reiterating that their response is of great value.

Teaching strategies questionnaire

The questionnaire was designed on a simple checklist approach, being easy to respond to and score (Tuckman, 1988). The teaching strategies were listed down the left-hand side of the page and the numbers 0 to 10 were put against each strategy.

For example:

Buzz Groups   0 1 2 3 4 5 6 7 8 9 10

The stem instructed the respondent to circle how many times they had undertaken that strategy within the last two weeks, in the classroom setting only. An example was given as part of the stem: 'Please note the number and type of strategies are independent of the number of sessions: For example in one teaching session I may use buzz groups twice, a lecture format once and group work once'. Feedback indicated that respondents found this helpful.

Using a checklist approach may mean that data are limited and elicit few opinions, therefore it was decided to leave two additional spaces for the respondents to add other teaching strategies they may have used and a space for comments which was open to interpretation. The respondents were given three weeks to complete and return the questionnaire and a request for comments on the letter orientation was included.

A key potential problem was the respondents' interpretation of what was meant by the named teaching strategy. In order to reduce variable interpretations and maintain rigour, a list of definitions was drawn up from a variety of authors (Bligh, 1971; Muir, 1984; English National Board, 1987; Jarvis, 1988; Thomson, 1988) and enclosed with the questionnaire.

A further problem was that the number of strategies used would be dependent to an extent of the opportunities for teaching, i.e. the number of teaching sessions within the last two weeks. Therefore the questionnaire format needed to ensure that each teacher stated the overall number of teaching sessions undertaken.

Caution is needed when using questionnaires, as respondents may say what they think is desirable or wanted by the researcher (Tuckman, 1988), however Kolb (1984) and Honey and Mumford (1992) say that self-perception of behaviours tends to be accurate providing the reason for data collection is not threatening.

The strategy definitions meant that they could be considered on a teacher-centred to student-centred continuum and with the increasing emphasis and popularity of the student-centred approach there was a potential reluctance for teachers to say they had used teacher-centred rather than student-centred activities. Therefore, when designing the questionnaire the strategies were deliberately intermingled and the wording very carefully considered in order to reduce such potential bias. A key point here is to trust one's instincts – I could not prove that the respondents would be reluctant to state that they had used teacher-centred activities but I considered that they would and therefore took this into consideration when planning the questionnaire format.

Using the same tool for this study could be criticized, though two factors can be said to support the decision. The first is that one of the limitations of correlation research data collection is that asking different things on the same tool can provide spurious correlation (Anderson, 1990) so using two different questionnaires could be justified. The second supporting factor is that having two questionnaires produced by different authors could reduce the risk of such inaccurate correlation.

Pilot

In order to gain data from people similar to the main population but not part of it (Parahoo and Reid, 1988), midwifery teachers (n = 13) were used to pilot the teaching strategies questionnaire. The pilot revealed that the term teaching session had been interpreted variably and comments were made on its ambiguity. This sentence was then revised and simplified. The 'last 10 working days' also proved ambiguous and was changed to 'your last 10 working days'. Quizs/tests had been used by the midwives, therefore this category was added to the questionnaire and to the list of definitions. Some criticism was made of not 'backing' the questionnaire thereby wasting paper. However, this practice was adhered to because it facilitated the respondent in using the guidance in the stem on the first page. The data revealed that some teachers used a wide range of strategies whereas others showed a definite emphasis towards strategies linked with a particular learning style.

At this point researchers must be willing to seriously consider whether to continue with the study as planned. One must be very certain that the data would be useful and valid. The results of the pilot study indicated that teachers would tend to use those strategies they are comfortable with (Bennett, 1976; Shaw, 1985; Honey and Mumford, 1992).

An issue did arise out of these data which I had not given sufficient consideration to: how to weight the teaching strategies according to the amount of sessions available to the teachers. After much arithmetical angst, a weighted percentage approach was used and the help of a person with a thorough understanding of statistics at this stage was vital.

Deciding on when a teaching strategy matches a learning style

In order to undertake the correlation exercise it was necessary to determine which teaching strategies 'linked' with which learning style (Figure 9.2). Based on the hypothesis that learning styles will influence teaching strategies each of the four learning style preferences could be said to have strategies that match. The decision on the categories was based on a variety of authors' work, but mostly that of Kolb (1984) and Honey and Mumford (1992).

There was a large degree of agreement about which teaching strategies suited which learning styles, the only area for argument being Kolb's (1984) statement that active experimenters (activists) liked to be self-directed while Honey and Mumford (1992) stated that activists learn least/dislike working alone so it depended upon the interpretation of whether self-directed

Activist

Role play
Games
Brainstorm
Self-directed (open learning)
Buzz groups
Workshops

Pragmatist

Care planning/care studies
Demonstrations
Simulations/practicals
Group discussion

Reflector

Films/videos/
Cassettes/slides
Guided discussion
Lecture
Guided study

Theorist

Computer-assisted programmes
Seminar
Quiz/tests
Tutorial
Debate

Figure 9.2 Learning styles and associated teaching strategies

means working alone. Although not synonymous the decision was to place self-directed in the activist domain.

A consistent problem when using the literature to designate teaching strategies to learning styles was that Fry (1977), Kolb (1984) and Honey and Mumford (1992) all tend not to identify teaching strategies theorists would find conducive to learning. Therefore acitivities related to the theorist learning style were designated by interpreting the learning preferences outlined by the authors.

On a teacher-centred/student-centred continuum a point for further discussion was that reflector activities tended to be teacher-centred whereas activist and pragmatist were student-centred strategies; theorist activities appeared to be a mix. Dux (1989) states that experiential methods correlate well with pragmatist preferences; however, the term experiential had been avoided when deciding on these categories. The rationale was the difficulty in terminology: experiential activities can be based on students' real experiences or can be teacher-generated imaginary situations (Thomson, 1988). Thus pragmatists preferring real application would not necessarily like or use experiential activities such as role play, whereas activists will enjoy and benefit from such strategies (providing there is not a lengthy reflection!). An important issue which affected the validity of this crucial part of the study was that all designated strategies could be implemented at any point on the teacher/student-centred continuum (English National

Board, 1987); while this is acknowledged the definitions sought to clarify the emphasis of student or teacher 'control' for each strategy.

Results

Learning style questionnaire

Of the 59 questionnaires returned only three were invalid, one because of total non-compliance and two because they were incomplete. Formal and informal feedback revealed that the questions were felt to be context dependent, i.e. that the behaviours changed according to circumstance which the questionnaire does not allow for, however Honey and Mumford (1992) do stress that the questionnaire is designed to reveal general tendencies.

Scoring the results is undertaken using the score key provided which by totalling the number of ticks in each column, a raw score is produced for each teacher. Although general norms are available Honey and Mumford (1992) recommend using the occupational norms in order fully to interpret the results into bands indicating strength of preference. The five bands range from very low preference to very strong preference; 15 of the 60 teachers who responded showed no strong or very strong preference. Dux (1989) states that this infers two possible causes: either that the respondent is too selective when answering the questionnaire or they had a low interest in learning. The latter was hopefully not the case!

Only 22.8 per cent of the teachers showed up as balanced learners, in that they benefited from new learning experiences and were adaptable. If one of the goals of education is to develop a range of learning skills in our students then this may require closer inspection. Teachers do use a variety of strategies but it could be argued that in order to develop such skills in students teachers must develop their own learning skills (Jarvis, 1992). The data were examined to see if gender or subject specialism affected preferences, but there were no clear tendencies seen. A key point here is that with quantitative data one can become more involved with number crunching than in keeping to the original purpose, but time spent checking possible trends/implications is worthwhile.

Reflectors were one of the two dominant learning styles in the Faculty (42.8 per cent). These are said to have particular strengths in the collection and analysis of information, both raw data and others' opinions (Honey and Mumford, 1992), these skills could be considered highly appropriate for an effective teaching and learning environment. The second dominant learning style was that of pragmatists who are essentially practical, and it would be expected that the nurse teachers would wish to apply knowledge to patient care, including the emphasis on applying new knowledge, i.e. research and problem solving which should enhance the learning environment.

An area of interest arose when analysing the data and considering Kolb's learning orientations and the links made with occupational choice/influence. The data indicated that when compared with the general norms the nurse teachers had more equivalence to assimilator rather than diverger, divergers being more people-orientated persons associated with nursing. Assimilators are associated with less practical pursuits, and more on an abstract dimension. These data would indicate that the teachers had 'moved away' from a style consistent with nursing. Hodges (1988) states that individuals tend to gravitate towards environments consistent with their personal characteristics, so one inference could be that this is why teachers leave clinical areas and ongoing patient contact. An alternative conclusion is that as environments are said to socialize contiguity between styles and environment then teachers within the Faculty have changed/adapted since being in the teaching environment. Honey and Mumford's questionnaire (1992) may have grown out of Kolb's work (1984) but drawing conclusions such as those put forward is too simplistic and would require further investigation.

Honey and Mumford (1992) place nurse teachers and nurses within the activist/reflector quadrant based on a comparison with all the occupational means. The results would indicate that the Faculty teachers were more representative of sixth form teachers/lecturers in the reflector/theorist quadrant than nurses/nurse teachers.

Teaching strategy questionnaire

If the hypothesis had been correct then according to the learning style questionnaire results the teachers would have reported more use of lectures, guided discussions and study with the use of films, etc. A broad range of activities would have been expected with less emphasis on student-centred activities of role play, brainstorming, etc. In quantitative research it is important not to forget the simple approach, so a straightforward addition process was undertaken. Of the 37 questionnaires returned activist strategies were the most frequent, followed by pragmatist, then reflector and with theorist occurring the least. These results were influenced by the fact that the strategies in the activist domain are short in time therefore likely to be more numerous.

The results of the questionnaires were scrutinized to see if teachers had used all strategies defined in the questionnaire and this was so. The weighted percentages incurred even more problems in that the smaller the number of teaching sessions the more likely that the results were non-typical.

On further examination of the figures and the range of strategies per teacher only four teachers seemed to use relatively 'similar' amounts of all four categories. Interestingly, two of the four teachers' results indicated that they had a balanced approach to learning. However, this relationship was not found elsewhere and so although worthy of note it could not be considered significant. A further point gained from the data was that over half (52.7 per cent) did not use the strategies linked with a particular learning style, so although the students received a broad range of teaching strategies if students had certain teachers consistently then some students did not receive strategies compatible with their learning style.

A point for consideration: the skills of the learner with a strong or very strong preference for reflector learning style appear to mirror some of the skills of reflective practice yet the teaching strategies that suit reflectors are considered to be teacher-centred. Rejection of teacher-guided activities may mean that students are not being helped to develop the very skills wanted of a practitioner. Although a tentative and tenuous link, this would merit further investigation and consideration.

Interpretation using Pearson Product Moment Coefficient

The use of the equation requires the use of a good calculator and patience and having identified the results of:

Activist:	r = plus	0.2776
Reflector:	r = minus	0.2332
Theorist:	r = plus	0.1175
Pragmatist:	r = plus	0.1043

then the significance and meaningfulness of the results needs thought and reflection. Values of 0.20 to 0.35 are considered to have limited meaning in exploratory work such as this (Cohen and Manion, 1989) and as this interpretation is based on analysis of 100 or more subjects and does not discuss factors of less than 0.2 then there was no presumable relationship. A further check against the probability values for Pearson's r (Clegg, 1982) showed that the level of significance was not even minimal. The coefficient of determination r^2 was used to specify how much of the variation in the predicted variable is due to the relationship with the other variable (Harper, 1991); this part of the analysis would have been of benefit if a high positive or negative correlation had been found.

Recommendations

The following comments are drawn from the experience of undertaking the study:

- note that undertaking correlation research may require you to use the same data resource twice, a point to consider with the subjects' patience;

- you may start with an adequate number in your sample but this diminishes rapidly and this needs to be considered when deciding on your original sample size;
- the data analysis will reveal the unexpected. This may seem a truism but needs to be included within the analysis and interpretation;
- you have to acknowledge the limitations of such number crunching when dealing with human beings;
- you have to consider how to reduce the variables very carefully as even limited significance can diminish. One of my suggestions for this study was to examine the teachers with different student groups in the same classroom and with the same subject area being taught;
- threat is still perceived despite the reassurance of confidentiality. Some of the teachers were defensive or apologetic about the teaching strategies they used, particularly when reporting the use of apparently teacher-centred strategies;
- quantitative research will have a distinct element of qualitative analysis and this could be considered to be one of its strengths;
- get actively involved in research. Undertaking this study through all the stages of the research process has to be one of the greatest leaps in learning I've ever experienced. Such learning can be a painful process but my teaching skills improved, my ability to examine the work of others increased and I have more insight into students' learning needs. Rather like buying a house – fraught during the process, great when you finally move in and then you discover all the work that is still to be done!

Conclusion

The results of the study were unequivocal, yet it does not disprove a relationship between teachers' learning styles and their choice of teaching strategies. The results may be more an indication of the design limitations, the use of self-reporting for both variables and the multifactorial nature of classroom teaching. The value of the study may include the designation of the categories of teaching strategies to learning styles, and the eminent authors' statements on what teaching methods are said to be most beneficial for the preferred learning style/s which have tended to be accepted uncritically. Drawing from their work the classification contributes to the debate about matching or mismatching teaching approaches and I hope other teachers will examine and citicize the proposed categorization of teaching strategies to the four learning styles. Combined with Sutcliffe's (1993) work on whether students change their learning style dependent upon the subject being studied, this could form the basis for a more in-depth examination of how we can facilitate effective learning for the students.

The move of nurse education provision into higher education institutions does have a considerable influence on curricula and so on the students' learning. The influence of teachers on the teaching/learning environment may become more visible with the advent of the subject grouping approach where potentially all students attend units which belong to specific subject groups and are taught by teachers with that subject specialism. The study does, however, indicate that teachers may not use any of the strategies that are suggested to benefit a certain learning style, it may therefore be possible that some students would not receive any teaching methods that are compatible with their preferred learning style.

However, the results of the teaching strategies questionnaire strongly indicated that most teachers within the Faculty used a wide range of methods and that the calls for a student-centred, progressive approach to teaching nurses have been answered. The challenge will be to maintain this development in these times of constricting resources and increasing demands, while not losing the breadth and variety of teaching strategies that are now available to the students.

Questionnaires can be a very useful and valid way of gaining data but should only be utilized when the research question and design require their use. I would recommend Oppenheim's (1992) edition for any researcher even considering the use of questionnaires in a study. However, it is as important to reflect upon questionnaires you have been asked to complete in the past, and remember what encouraged their completion. As with any data collection tool, questionnaires can enhance or detract from the usefulness of a study and the element of researcher-bias should not be underestimated. As questionnaires are often used for student evaluation of units and courses, it may be a profitable exercise to re-examine your own establishment's forms and consider if they are an effective measurement tool.

Learning styles are an interesting concept and identification of preferences can be of great personal use. I do, however, have qualms about their use in nurse education and the studies (including mine) which claim to have identified students' and staff learning preferences. The main concern is that data should be used for the benefit of the respondents; we do not help students if we claim to utilize the learning style information as a basis for our teaching and then ignore or forget it for the rest of their programme. The second is that the data must be used carefully. Honey and Mumford (1992) stress that students need to be made aware that learning style preferences can be changed for the better, i.e. what one is said to be good at or bad at can become a self-fulfilling prophecy if it is not dealt with skilfully. This is one reason why I recommend that you return to the original works by Honey and Mumford and Kolb but read widely on the significance of learning styles, Schmeck's book (1988) is very helpful in showing the differing perspectives.

Unless you have undertaken a statistics course recently, the help of a knowledgeable colleague is vital when undertaking quantitative research. Each study has unique characteristics but it is very important that statistical advice is sought early in the research process as the planned data collection may be inappropriate to the statistical analysis. I used my contacts to access help which was given freely in monetary terms and time; however, professional assistance can be obtained at a cost and computer packages are available (the local college and library should be able to assist). I found that books on statistics tended either to try and cover everything and were too simplistic or so complex that one needed a course to understand the book! However, re-reading some of the basics is essential prior to seeking advice or you may not understand the nuances of the guidance.

Quantitative research has its supporters and critics, and to some extent it has now been rejected by nurses as too mechanistic and indicative of a return to our past research efforts. However, the data are concrete, visible and open to scrutiny, aspects that qualitative research does not always possess. More controversially, nurses and nurse teachers are in the midst of a struggle to prove that they have academic credibility and research expertise equivalent to other professions. Proof of this may have to be determined by hard data which can be reproduced and tested. Whatever methods are used, maintaining rigour through an explicit theoretical underpinning, considering the use of triangulation and a meticulous approach to writing the research report is essential.

Research is an activity which teachers will have to consider as part of their everyday working lives and as necessary as lesson preparation. Making time and having prepared for hard work are key requirements but it does not always have to be serious, it can even be fun!

Acknowledgement

With thanks to Dr Peter Honey for his permission to publish.

References

Anderson G (1990) *Fundamentals of Educational Research.* Falmer Press, London.

Bennett N (1976) *Teaching Style and Pupil Progress.* Open Books, London.

Bligh D A (1971) *What's the Use of Lectures?* Bligh & Bligh, Exeter.

Clegg F (1982) *Simple Statistics: A Course Book for the Social Sciences.* Cambridge University Press, Cambridge.

Cohen L and Manion L (1989) *Research Methods in Education*, 3rd edn. Routledge, London.

Dunn R S and Dunn K J (1979) Learning styles: should they . . . can they . . . be matched? *Educational Leadership* 36 (4) January, 238–44.

Dux C M (1989) An investigation into whether nurse teachers take into account the individual learning styles of their students when formulating teaching strategies. *Nurse Education Today* 9 (3), 186–91.

English National Board (1987) *Managing Change in Nursing Education*. ENB, London.

Fry R (1977) Diagnosing professional learning environments: an observational framework for matching learning styles with types of situational complexity. PhD Dissertation, Sloan School of Management, Institute of Technology.

Harper W M (1991) *Statistics*, 6th edn. Longman, London.

Hodges S A (1988) Individual learning styles of student nurses, their teachers and ward sisters. *Journal of Advanced Nursing* 13 (3), 341–4.

Honey P and Mumford A (1992) *The Manual of Learning Styles*. Honey, Maidenhead.

Jarvis P (1988) *Adult and Continuing Education: Theory and Practice*. Routledge, London.

Jarvis P (1992) Quality in practice: the role of education. *Nurse Education Today* 12 (1), 3–10.

Joyce C R B and Hudson L (1968) Student style and teacher style: an experimental study. *British Journal of Medical Education* 2, 28–32.

Kolb D A (1984) *Experiential Learning: Experience as the Source of Learning and Development*. Prentice-Hall, Englewood Cliffs.

Lapeyre E (1992) Nursing students' learning styles: a comparison of degree and non-degree student approaches to studying. *Nurse Education Today* 12 (3), 192–9.

Laschinger S, Ogden Burke S and Jerret M (1986) Teaching styles: is the modular method more effective? *Nursing Papers/Perspectives on Nursing* 18 (4), 15–25.

Macleod Clark J and Hockey L (1979) *Research for Nursing*. HM&M, Aylesbury.

McMillan M A and Dwyer J (1990) Facilitating a match between teaching and learning styles. *Nurse Education Today* 10 (3), 186–92.

Oppenheim A N (1992) *Questionnaire Design, Interviewing and Attitude Measurement*, 2nd edn. Pinter, London.

Parahoo K and Reid N (1988) Research skills. Number 2. *Nursing Times* 84 (5), 67–70.

Partridge R (1983) Learning styles: a review of selected models. *Journal of Nursing Education* 22 (6), 243–8.

Schmeck R R (Ed.) (1988) *Learning Strategies and Learning Styles*. Plenum Press, London.

Shaw D G (1985) Preparing students to be health educators. Masters Dissertation (M Ed.), University of London.

Sutcliffe L (1993) An investigation into whether nurses change their learning style according to subject area studied. *Journal of Advanced Nursing* 18 (4) 647–58.

Thomson A J (1988) The effects of preparation on the practice of teaching. Masters Dissertation (M Ed.), Institute of Education, University of London.

Tuckman B W (1988) *Conducting Educational Research*, 3rd edn. Harcourt Brace Jovanovich, London.

10

A matter of degree: factors influencing a teacher's pursuit of degree studies

Val Smith

In this chapter the rationale for implementation of a critique of a survey is discussed in depth. Reading this chapter will offer you many useful insights and pitfalls to avoid. Most students new to research have heard of this approach:

- *the literature review clearly weighs the argument towards the need for a survey;*
- *the rationale advantages and disadvantages of this method are outlined and lead towards an argument for the approach adopted;*
- *there are clear lessons to be learned on questionnaire design;*
- *presentation of the findings demonstrates the value of this method with the contrast of tables and discussion.*

Introduction

The research project described in this chapter was submitted in May 1991 in part fulfilment of the requirements for a Bachelor of Arts (Honours) degree in Nursing Education, awarded by the University of Manchester. The study forms an exploration of the factors which determine nurse and midwife teachers' reasons for pursuing degree qualifications. In addition to presenting the research undertaken, a discussion on the use of the survey as a research method is included. Personal 'hands-on' experience is drawn upon to highlight the advantages and disadvantages of the use of the survey as a research method.

Successes and failures encountered on the way are discussed in the hope that others starting out on research projects, without much previous experience, may gain some encouragement to continue when all is not going as smoothly as anticipated.

Throughout this chapter the word 'nurse' is used in its generic sense, unless otherwise specified. Similarly, the term 'teacher' is used to embrace all grades of tutor, teacher or lecturer practitioner.

Background to the study

The past decade has seen considerable change occurring both within the nursing profession and the National Health Service as a whole. For nurse education, the most significant of these innovations are contained in the radical reforms brought about by implementation of the Project 2000 proposals (RCN, 1985; UKCC, 1986).

One of the main intended outcomes of Project 2000 is to raise standards of nursing care by providing a high quality of education to pre-registration students. Nurse recruits who undertake Project 200 courses will follow programmes with a higher academic content and will qualify with a Diploma in Nursing. To this end, the UKCC also recommended that all teaching staff, in any field of nursing, should possess a degree (UKCC, 1987), thereby committing themselves to developing an all-graduate teaching profession. This, inter alia, aims to enhance academic credibility in the nursing profession.

If nurse teaching is to become an all-graduate profession it will have financial, manpower and resource implications for individual teaching staff, their colleagues, the educational institutions employing them and those institutions offering degree courses. Some salient questions need to be addressed and include the following:

- Who will benefit from an all-graduate teaching profession in nursing?
- What is meant by a degree?
- What level of degree will be required?
- Should the degree taken be related to nursing?
- Who will fund staff undertaking degrees?
- What study leave will be given?
- What provision will be made to cover work-loads while staff are taking study leave?
- What do individual staff feel about an all-graduate teaching profession in nursing?
- Will nursing be able to recruit sufficient teachers with degree status?
- Will there be financial, or other rewards when the degree has been gained?
- How many teaching staff already possess degrees?
- What will happen to those staff already qualified as nurse teachers who do not wish to undertake degree studies?
- What are the overall implications in the management of the growing numbers of nurse and midwife teachers undertaking degrees?

The list of questions is not meant to be exhaustive. It merely seeks to give some indication of the issues involved and some idea of those background areas requiring further consideration. The concept of an all-graduate teaching profession in nursing is a new innovation for teacher preparation and, as such, must be classed as a major change.

These were some of my initial thoughts when first contemplating what the Project 2000 proposals would mean for the individual practitioner, the nursing profession as a whole and the potential benefits, or otherwise, for the recipients of the service. The topic of degree studies was of relevance because of the degree course I was undertaking. However, the implications that all teachers should possess degrees put much greater emphasis on the enormity of the proposals for individual professional development and for the profession overall. My personal interest in this area stemmed primarily from these proposals.

While studying for a degree, significant reorganization was taking place within my own workplace. In common with many other educational establishments, individual midwifery and nursing schools were responding to ENB recommendations by amalgamating to form large Colleges of Nursing and Midwifery. Links were also being forged with the Higher Education sector.

At the micro level I perceived that there was an increase in the number of midwife teachers undertaking degree studies from what seemed to be approximately 25 per cent in 1986 to around 50 per cent in 1989. This led to development of the hypothesis which forms the basis for this research study and which is discussed after the literature review.

Literature review

A search of the available British literature on nurse and midwife educators and their attitudes to enhancing professional credibility by possessing degrees, revealed that this was an apparently neglected field. Similarly, in reviewing the literature on attitudes towards continued professional development, only a limited amount of material was available relating specifically to teaching staff. The search was therefore extended to embrace literature on the motivation of post-registered nursing professionals to continue their education and development as all teachers would have gone through initial nurse education programmes followed by a period of practice (UKCC, 1988).

A dearth of information on continuing education among British nurses was available prior to the mid-1980s, most of the material coming through recently. Therefore, reference was also made to the more extensive literature available in North America, although it is important to remember that cultural differences between American and British nursing may affect outcomes.

Research undertaken by Rogers and Lawrence (1986) in the United

Kingdom focused on the continuing education of qualified nurses. It revealed that, when support and interest from senior colleagues was available and evident to the sample interviewed, the likelihood of them becoming involved in continuing professional education was enhanced. However, the study also highlighted a considerable gulf between the commitment expressed by health authorities towards continuing education and the extent to which this commitment was actually demonstrated in practice.

More recent literature (Rogers, 1987; Carlisle, 1991) would indicate that the role of the employing health authorities still requires scrutiny as the provision of continuing education varies considerably, with some authorities providing wide-ranging opportunities and others very little. Similarly, a lack of commitment to continuing education by those managing the nursing services has been identified by both Chiarella (1990) and Ward (1990) as de-motivators for those wishing to continue their education after qualifying.

The reforms to the National Health Service (DoH, 1989a, 1989b), indicate that health authorities will need to ensure that the services provided are cost effective yet still manage to deliver a high standard of care. Furthermore, the DoH has confirmed that future funding for pre- and post-registration nurse and midwifery education will be devolved to the regional health authorities, while in-service education remains the responsibility of individual employers. Educational institutions will also be required to demonstrate similar cost effectiveness. This may introduce a dichotomy between colleges which are trying to provide academic excellence and the providers of health care who may be financially constrained. In an area where cost-cutting and financial implications are already being felt, continuing professional education may well become the poor relation.

It appears that non-postgraduate courses and study days may only be provided for qualified staff if these courses generate significant funds for educational institutions, rather than to increase the knowledge and skills of the professional! If the UKCC (1987) is serious in its intentions to develop an all-graduate profession then these are important factors requiring further consideration.

The professional nursing body of the United Kingdom demonstrated its commitment to encourage practitioners to improve their professional knowledge after qualifying when it published the Code of Professional Conduct (UKCC, 1984). This linked accountability and competence to continuing education and put responsibility for updating firmly with the individual. This commitment is solidly reinforced by the recommendations contained in the consultation document on Post-registration Education and Professional Practice, PREPP, (UKCC, 1990). The proposed minimum of five days mandatory refreshment every three years for *all* practitioners may well affect the way practitioners perceive the importance of continuing education and, subsequently, their overall motivation.

Popiel (1969), in discussing continuing education in American nursing, highlighted several factors likely to motivate professionals to undertake further study. These were to gain knowledge in order to practise more efficiently, to learn new nursing skills, to boost self-development and professional growth and because mandatory re-licensure required evidence of additional learning.

A later American study by O'Connor (1979), examined the relationship between nurses' motivation for participation in mandatory continuing education with their motivation when it was non-legislative. It concluded that nurses were more likely to participate in order to improve practice rather than because of legislation. These findings have been substantiated in further work carried out by Faulkenberry (1986), Urbano (1988) and de Haven (1990). It will be interesting to see the extent to which nurse and midwife teachers are likely to be influenced by the statutory graduate status proposed in the United Kingdom.

Millonig (1985) investigated some of the links between the concept of professionalism, continuing education and adult learning. Her findings suggest that continual learning is not promoted sufficiently, making subsequent choices for further study difficult. However, concurring with Popiel (1969), she concludes that nurses participated in continuing education for a number of reasons including: to earn a degree or other certificate, to obtain higher status in their jobs, to secure professional advancement and to maintain, or improve, their social position. This work is backed up in the United Kingdom in a recent study undertaken by Mackereth (1989).

Studdy and Hunt (1980), Altschul (1982) and Lahiff (1983), however, have all argued that some practitioners do not perceive that they have a responsibility towards maintaining their own educational needs and suggest it is important for employing authorities to be more explicit in their commitment to continuing education.

Davidson (1991, p. 50) has stated that 'it is still possible for a nurse, once qualified, to avoid any brush with education for the rest of her career', while Brown (1988) doubts that mandatory professional updating will do much to motivate those 'laggards' who do not see the need to update themselves in order to improve practice. In addition, Rogers (1987) highlighted that even where the need to continue professional education had been identified, many obstacles were present to discourage practitioners who were keen to advance their own professional education and development.

Nugent (1990), in contrast, found that nurses were becoming increasingly aware of the need to continue education beyond initial registration and linked de-motivating factors to work hours, course availability and attitudes of nurses towards further study. Lathlean and Farnish (1984) demonstrated shortage of staff, lack of NHS finances and inadequate advance publicity as important factors mitigating against the uptake of continuing education. Mackereth (1989) and McCrea (1989) both discuss the effects of inappropriately applied learning methods and insufficient use of self-directed learning as additional factors. Sweeney (1986) also comments that some British nurses appear to be prejudiced both against the concepts underlying learner-centred education and the moves into academia.

Some of these studies may have parallels in the field of education where staff are already working under increasingly heavy workloads (Webster, 1990). Undertaking degree studies inevitably increases the overall work, both of the degree students taking part-time courses and their colleagues who may have to cover while they are away. This may discourage teachers contemplating higher education and decrease motivation significantly.

Among post-registered nurses, Kershaw (1990b) has stated that there is an increase in the numbers undertaking Open University courses to obtain degrees and that this trend is likely to grow. She also indicates that nurses seem to be reluctant to undertake higher education in establishments such as polytechnics or universities. If, indeed, there is a reluctance to obtain degrees in centres of higher education, this may be related to many of the factors influencing motivation which have already been discussed. It may also be due to the increased difficulty in gaining funding for further study (Carlisle, 1991; Friend, 1991). If these patterns are reflected in nurse teacher attitudes towards higher education, they may give valuable insights into the future develpment of an all-graduate teaching profession in nursing.

Although funding for nurse teacher preparation is primarily obtained through the ENB, the responsibility for its administration is devolved to individual health authorities (ENB, 1988). In a formal study, commissioned by the ENB examining nurse teacher preparation, Buttigieg (1990) has highlighted the many inconsistencies which exist in the interpretation of the Board's guidelines and the different levels of commitment between one health authority and another. Similarly, she also found that careers advice given to potential nurse teachers was haphazard and related more to local needs rather than the wider national issues. To some extent the implication is that local service and education requirements take precedence over any individual needs for professional development and the national requirements. Personal observation also suggests that this extends to those post-registered teachers wishing to further their academic education but no specific literature could be found to substantiate this claim.

Allan (1987, p. 211) demonstrates that in the last decade qualified nurse teachers have become increasingly aware of the need to continue educational studies beyond their initial teaching qualification. She states that 'In a study undertaken by the author in 1981 of nurses, midwives and health visitors holding a teaching qualification, it was shown that 34.5 per cent had undertaken additional education following their teaching qualifications'. Unfortunately, elucidation of what 'additional education' entailed was not given. Similarly, Kershaw (1990a, p. 4) quotes that 'over 50 per cent of present nurse teachers are already graduates or studying for degrees'.

Buttigieg (1990), in evaluating the preparation of teachers within nursing, midwifery and health visiting, estimated that 29.5 per cent of her sample already held, or were studying for, a degree (25.6 and 3.9 per cent respectively). Again from her cohort, 70.6 per cent intended studying for either a first, or higher degree, on completion of their teaching course. These statistics would imply that there is already a greater awareness among potential nurse teachers of the need to undertake further academic study.

In an earlier investigative study, relating specifically to midwife teachers, I also found a comparable figure (60 per cent) for those who possessed or were actively studying for a degree and that 32 per cent of the remainder intended to undertake degree studies within the following two years (Smith, 1990, unpublished). The study indicated that higher education was being pursued for reasons of personal growth and to broaden experience, motivation being intrinsic rather than extrinsic.

The information gained from the literature search has enabled me to put the subject of the research undertaken into context. Statistical evidence has shown that more nurse teachers are striving for graduate status. However, the lack of researched evidence on the motivating factors behind qualified nurse teachers undertaking degrees leaves this an open area for examination. Is the motivating factor a love of learning, to maintain personal professional development or an attempt by nurse teachers to further their careers? Conversely, does it merely indicate that it is the statutory nursing bodies and the educational institutions taking the lead rather than the individual practitioner, or is it due to a combination of factors?

Whether there is a relationship between the Project 2000 proposals and the increasing numbers of nurse teachers acquiring degrees remains to be seen. The research project outlined seeks to answer some of the questions posed and thereby identify some of the implications for future educational management.

The survey as a research method

Lancaster (1975) highlights that research methods can generally be classified under two broad headings, experimental and non-experimental or descriptive (commonly referred to as the survey). This differentiation may indicate that there are some advantages and disadvantages inherent in the use of the survey as a research method which must be borne in mind throughout the practical application of the research process. A working knowledge of these is invaluable to the researcher as they may significantly affect the way in which the research is conducted. In my own experience, a full understanding of the benefits and drawbacks of using the appropriate research method also helps to minimize the many pitfalls into which it is all too easy to fall.

McNeill (1985) maintains that use of the survey generally allows the researcher to proceed through the well-defined stages of the research process in an orderly manner, although the sequences may be varied slightly. This may be of particular benefit for the novice researcher as it provides useful guidelines to follow and facilitates a systematic approach when undertaking research. This structured approach was particularly useful for my own research both during the early planning stages and subsequently, as it helped to ensure that no stages of the research process were omitted.

Defining the purpose of the proposed piece of research (often the hardest part of the research project), reviewing the literature and then deciding what specific information is required will dictate which research method it is most appropriate to use. Further consideration can then be given to the size of the study, how the population is to be selected, what data are to be collected and how the data are to be analysed and presented. These aspects are comprehensively discussed by Abdellah and Levine (1979) who also expand on the importance of gathering data that are objective and to which measurement can be applied. Where the collated data do not allow statistical analysis to take place they maintain, as does McNeill (1985), that this type of research may well be denigrated.

Lancaster (1975) reveals that if a research proposal is well constructed, the researcher is likely to find it easier to obtain funding from outside sources. Furthermore, when the research is completed and the findings are presented, they will be more likely to be accepted and adopted. My own experience of not obtaining funding for earlier sociological research projects (not considerd 'scientific', or capable of generating controlled statistical data, by medical colleagues) would lead me to concur with these beliefs. Fortunately, more recent experiences show that colleagues are now a little more enlightened.

Cohen and Manion (1989) discuss fully the ways in which the survey approach lends itself well to the systematic observation of existing situations or events which can then be evaluated, explained and/or described. Its wide use for social science research is beneficial in providing answers to the questions of what happened where, when or how and to whom? Bell (1987) outlines that, unfortunately, it often has the disadvantage of not being able to answer the question of why, nor of determining causal relationships between events. Also, there is unlikely to be a unique interpretation of the results.

Abdellah and Levine (1979) highlight how the researcher often has little control over the conditions under which information is gathered as these are invariably of a personal or factual nature. Such studies frequently involve the use of human populations and it is all too easy to end up with a surfeit of data. On the other hand, if insufficient data are collected it will be difficult to present research from which valid and accurate inferences can be made. In order to achieve a balance between the two, it is necessary to determine carefully, in advance, which variables are to be employed.

Wilson (1975) expounds that variables have the advantage that they can help to eliminate many of the biases that could produce false data. Their choice and usefulness is dependent upon data sources and should be capable of demonstrating differences that can be measured statistically. Therefore, it is essential to consider choice of variables, techniques of data collection and selection of the study population in parallel. Abdellah and Levine (1979) both concur that if these elements are all taken into equal account, this helps to minimize the dangers that lead to misinterpretation of, or erroneously applied, causal relationships. Personally, I found the whole question of variables a difficult concept to comprehend and always have to battle with them. Subsequently, some problems occurred with my own research which are discussed later.

Cohen and Manion (1989) maintain that the survey allows large amounts of data to be collected in a relatively short period of time and, depending on the size of the study and the techniques used to gather information, need not incur vast expense. For many researchers time is often very limited and resources scant. Carelessness in selection of the survey population and inappropriate choice of the research instrument for data collection can waste valuable time and make the whole process unworkable. This was borne out in my own research and, again, is discussed later.

The population to be surveyed should be accessible, manageable and large enough accurately to represent the total population under review. Very large numbers can be studied, but this may render the project unwieldy and excessively expensive. For practical reasons, a representative sample of the total population is often used and achieved by the means of random sampling. If the characteristics of the sample population are truly representative of the whole, this allows for wider inferences and generalizations to be made from the research findings. The dangers of inappropriate selection of population sample are eloquently outlined by both Abdellah and Levine (1979) and Reid and Boore (1987).

These authors also discuss the techniques employed for gathering data which generally involve the use of questionnaires and/or interviews, although observation and attitude scales may also be incorporated. The information obtained should be able to withstand statistical analysis, from which patterns can be extracted and comparisons made between different populations.

NcNeill (1985) suggests that the main advantages of questionnaires over interviews are that larger numbers can be surveyed, they can be sent by post, administered in less time, at a lower cost, and anonymity of respondents can be assured. Also, because anonymity is maintained the information obtained is likely to be without personal bias and to have greater validity. However, the advantages must be set against the disadvantages that the response rates may be considerably lower and, later, information may be misinterpreted and it is not possible to elicit further responses from participants.

Much other useful information on the advantages and disadvantages of each method can be found in many of the texts already referenced. Practical application, however, is not always easy. My personal advice, hopefully to encourage the reader, would be for them to read widely around the topic and to accept any help proferred, or available, from any other source.

I found my own research supervisor particularly helpful here while also obtaining valuable advice and guidelines from my Regional Health Authority Nursing Research Department. Senior colleagues, with expertise in the research process, proved to be another invaluable source of information.

Once all the stages outlined above have been accomplished, all factors taken into consideration, pilot studies undertaken and tools for data collection refined, it only remains to collect the data, process and analyse the results, formulate conclusions and write up the results.

Embracing this in a single paragraph is not intended to imply that the final stages are less significant or less important than the earlier preparation. Rather, it is anticipated that presentation of my own research will link the process more clearly to the survey process and give greater direction/ meaning to the reader.

Research in action

As a relative novice in carrying out research methods, it soon became clear that, although I thought I had a fairly good grounding in the theoretical concepts underpinning the subject, practical application was a different matter. Many mistakes occurred due to sheer practical inexperience. Fortunately, advice and support from others with greater experience, coupled with unfailing encouragement from family, friends and work colleagues, meant that the research was finally completed, complied and submitted, albeit with some trepidation.

The research presented here extends earlier work which tested the same hypothesis, but studied a midwife population only. The main recommendations were that the study needed to be extended to validate results and widened to encompass both nurse and midwife teachers, in order to look at any inherent differences between cohorts.

Rationale for the choice of research method

The main aim of this research was to investigate the possible effects of one of the proposals contained in Project 2000 on the future career structure of qualified nurse and midwife educators. The research explores the factors which motivate nurse and midwife teachers to undertake degree studies. In parallel, it also seeks to answer some subsidiary questions which arose when defining the purpose of the study. These included:

- The opinions of nurse and midwife teachers on proposals that all qualified teachers in nursing should possess a degree.
- The extent to which nurse and midwife teachers already possess, or are currently studying for, a degree.
- The level of support available to nurse and midwife teachers undertaking degrees as opposed to the amount of support they feel should be available.
- Whether there are significant differences between nurse and midwife teacher populations.
- Possible implications for future educational management.

The hypothesis to be tested was that 'The apparent increase in the number of nurse and midwife teachers currently undertaking (or preparing to undertake) degree studies can be directly linked to the proposal contained in Project 2000 that all nurse and midwife teachers should possess a degree'.

Definition of the purpose of the study and subsequent literature review indicated that the topic under examination did not lend itself to the controlled, manipulative, conditions which are necessary for experimental research. The approach to be taken would involve studying a specific target population in order to generate sociological data which would portray an accurate picture of events at a given point in time. As such, this comes under the heading of non-experimental research.

To some extent, the subject area was determined by the degree I was undertaking. The final element of the course required the learner to present a dissertation. It was pre-specified that this would be related to the field of education while also demonstrating a working knowledge of the research process.

I needed to obtain information, in a specific topic area, which could be analysed relatively easily and quickly. Constraints on time were a major consideration as the complete process had to be undertaken, written up and presented by a specific date. Similarly, the question of financing and resources for the project needed to be addressed. I felt that it was unlikely that outside funding would be available, therefore data collection needed to keep costs to a minimum.

For the reasons outlined earlier, it became clear that the survey was the method of choice for this piece of research. The research presented forms a comparative study between nurse and midwife teachers, the general approach being that of a descriptive survey.

At the outset of the research project the expertise of a statistician was sought to give advice on the size of population needed to undertake a comphrehensive study and to give guidance on the most appropriate research tools likely to yield measurable results.

I was fortunate that I worked for an enlightened health authority, well versed in the need to encourage staff to undertake research. I also found that I was able to use the statistician employed by them and that this would not incur any financial outlay on my part. This was a great bonus for me and certainly reduced my apprehension levels on any matters statistical. Help from my husband was also invaluable along with two 'life-saving' texts, which I heartily recommend to anyone finding themselves in a similar position of statistical illiteracy: Wilson (1975) and Swinscow (1980).

A population size of 60 was accepted as being sufficiently large to generate valid results, but not so large as to be unmanageable or incur unnecessary expense. In order to enable comparisons to be made between groups, I aimed to obtain responses from an equal number of nurse and midwife teachers.

The nurse teacher population was selected from a College of Health Care Studies, recently formed following amalgamation of three schools of nursing and four schools of midwifery. Because of the size of the college, it was decided that the whole nurse teacher cohort could be obtained from the one institution.

The midwife teacher cohort was retained from the earlier study undertaken by me in the previous year. Two-thirds of this cohort came from the same College of Health Care Studies as the nurse teacher cohort. The remaining third were recruited from another college with similar characteristics. Both colleges had undergone significant reorganization within the previous 12 months.

Because the number of nurse teachers in any combined College of Nursing and Midwifery is likely to outweight the number of midwife teachers the cohort of nurse teachers was randomly selected. This approach was taken to gain a representative sample of the nurse teacher population. A simple systematic random sample, as recommended by Best (1981), was made using every third nurse teacher from an alphabetical list. This was maintained by the college personnel department. No such luxury was available for selecting midwives because of the vastly smaller numbers.

The nurse and midwife teachers all met the same criteria for inclusion in the study. All were qualified to teach in their particular speciality (i.e. nursing or midwifery) and all were actively involved in teaching. No distinction was made between levels of responsibility in the college hierarchy (educational grade). This decision was made to enable an overall picture of degree study to emerge. It would also allow comparisons to be made between levels of responsibility and attitudes towards the possession of degrees.

I had some qualms about using the same respondents from an earlier study and including their responses in the current research. However, as the hypothesis and research method were exactly the same for both studies my research advisor and the statistician felt that this would not render the results invalid. Participants in the original cohort were all followed up to check their current status, especially with regard to their degree courses. The original data obtained from this group were acquired only six months prior to the research presented.

Funding for the research project had been requested from my immediate employers but, unfortunately, this was not granted. Perhaps if more time had been available to complete the research, I could have planned more strategically and approached several other sources which may have been interested in funding such a project. For example, I could have approached the regional health authority or The King's Fund Centre, or submitted an application to one of the educational, charitable or pharmaceutical organizations which generously provide scholarships for those wishing to undertake research (e.g. the Edwina Mountbatten Trust, the Iolanthe Trust, The Smith and Nephew Foundation).

The research was undertaken using postal questionnaires and semi-structured interviews. The rationale for this was to obtain both quantitative and qualitative data, thus providing more information than would have been obtained by use of one technique alone.

The use of a questionnaire format was also made because it provided a reasonably simple and inexpensive method of data collection, it allowed information to be gathered fairly rapidly, preserved the anonymity of the respondents and is recommended as an appropriate tool to use for survey research by many of the authors already referenced.

The questionnaire was designed in two sections, following a format recommended by Oppenheim (1966). The first section consisted of a series of questions which were structured to elicit demographic details, to explore the extent to which nurse and midwife teachers were undertaking degree studies and to examine motivational factors.

Fox (1976) suggests that the success of a questionnaire is likely to be greater if early questions are non-threatening. These can then be followed by more in-depth questions requiring more highly structured answers or opinions. Similarly, my questionnaire design also ensured that initial questions were relatively easy to score with latter questions requiring more thought. The questionnaire was pre-coded (as advised by Cohen and Manion, 1989) and consisted almost entirely of closed questions. Pre-coding ensured that confidentiality and anonymity of the respondent was assured throughout the study.

The second section of the questionnaire was designed to highlight the different attitudes and beliefs of the two cohorts towards degree study in nurse and midwifery education. Although the attitude scale was not easy to design it proved to be a valuable tool as it generated very worthwhile data.

The questionnaire was piloted using a representative sample (20 per cent) of the original cohort. The pilot study was undertaken to test the validity and reliability of the questionnaire and to ensure that data collected were suitable for analysis. This resulted in some questions being omitted because of similarities between questions or because the information did not yield material relevant to the study. Other questions required re-organization to enable the questionnaire to follow a logical sequence, or re-wording to achieve greater clarity.

Even though questionnaires were piloted twice, subsequent reflection on the findings of the research indicated that one of the questions was not entirely relevant to the study and could have been omitted. Fortunately, the extraneous matter obtained did not affect final outcomes but the extra work involved in analysis was onerous. Similarly, two other questions would have benefited from further refinement to generate more sophisticated data. It is difficult to estimate, in retrospect, whether a further pilot study on the nurse population would have picked up these discrepancies. These are discussed later in the chapter.

Questionnaires were posted during the week before Christmas. A specific, short duration return date, as recommended by Cohen and Manion (1989), was set in order to increase the likelihood of a good response. An explanatory letter accompanied the questionnaire giving details of the research project and requesting participants' cooperation. A message was also attached to the questionnaires indicating that a 100 per cent return rate would be a wonderful Christmas and New Year present for the author. These two strategies resulted in the very gratifying response rate of 100 per cent. Many responses also contained good luck messages, indicating that several of the cohort had obviously undergone similar experiences! I am also aware that the response rate was possibly influenced by my personally knowing many of the teachers and this is also acknowledged.

Cohen and Manion (1989, p. 114) state that 'A well-planned postal survey should obtain at least a 40 per cent response rate and with the judicious use of reminders, a 70 per cent to 80 per cent response level should be possible'. NcNeill (1985, p. 36) quotes similar figures of 30–40 per cent response rates for postal questionnaires. I therefore consider myself extremely fortunate in obtaining the outstanding response rates which I achieved.

In addition to the questionnaire a proportion of the cohort were also interviewed. This was accomplished by random sampling, as recommended by Best (1981), every fifth person from the questionnaire code being included. In order to minimize bias all interviews were conducted by myself. These were informal, restricted to 30 minutes and took place in the individual teacher's office. Confidentiality was stressed to enable colleagues to express themselves without fear of being quoted, or information being used against them.

A semi-structured interview format was chosen to explore participants' views about nurse and midwife teachers gaining degree status and to clarify any points that were unclear from the questionnaires. Notes were taken during the interview and written up within 24 hours of the interview taking place. Best (1981) and Cohen and Manion (1989) give many useful tips on interview techniques which I did incorporate, but I wish that I had also accepted the recommendation to record interviews on tape.

The interview component was very time-consuming, both in terms of conducting the interview and in analysing and making sense of the data afterwards. It is not a strategy to be embarked on lightly! Possibly the same results could have been achieved using a different technique, such as including a section for extended comments on the questionnaire.

Prior to data analysis questionnaires were checked for completeness and accuracy, after which the data were reduced and fed into the appropriate computer spreadsheet which was self-designed. Perhaps use of a statistical package, such as the Statistical Package for the Social Sciences (Nie *et al.*, 1975), would have rendered this task a little less time consuming.

Data analysis of Section A of the questionnaire was mainly quantitative. Where appropriate and where group sizes allowed, the standard Chi-squared analyses were conducted. The question exploring motivation for undertaking degree study was analysed using a quantitative weighted ranking analyses. Analysis of Section B was undertaken using Likert-type scales in order to quantify responses on attitudes to degree study. I found the texts of Swinscow (1980) and Best (1981) were particularly valuable for this. Data from the semi-structured interview were analysed using both quantitative and qualitative methods. The latter involved the use of a modified grounded-theory approach as described by Glaser and Strauss (1967).

The information gained from data analysis is presented to form a logical sequence, not in the order that questions were asked. Data from the questionnaire are presented first and supported with information acquired from the semi-structured interviews. This should allow demographic details of age and educational background to emerge, followed by a picture of current educational activities, the amount of support available and the motivating factors for undertaking degree studies.

Findings of the attitude survey are considered as a separate entity to highlight the different attitudes and beliefs towards degree study and continued professional education. This should allow a discussion to emerge on the different expectations of nurse and midwife teachers and what happens in reality. A comparison between midwife and nurse teacher responses is made throughout, along with an estimation of their relevance to the research findings.

Findings

Age

Ages for both midwife teachers and nurse teachers ranged between 25 and 64 years (Table 10.1). Against all expectations, the midwife teacher group appeared to qualify as teachers at an earlier age than their nurse teacher

Table 10.1   Age spread of midwife and nurse teacher cohorts

Years	RMT cohort (30)		RNT cohort (30)	
	No.	%	No.	%
25–34	9	30	2	7
35–44	9	30	14	47
45–54	9	30	10	33
Over 55	3	10	4	13

RMT = Midwife teachers; RNT = Nurse teachers for all the tables in this chapter. Percentages have been rounded to the nearest integer throughout.

colleagues. Since all the midwife teachers in the cohort possessed a first-level nursing qualification, in addition to being qualified midwives, it seemed a reasonable assumption to expect them to be older. No specific conclusions were made to explain this difference. The findings may be purely incidental and a much wider, more sophisticated study would need to be conducted to reveal if there is any significance.

Professional and teaching qualifications

This question generated a vast amount of data which were difficult to quantify. The intention had been to identify whether there were any patterns of study leading to graduate status. However, as the year for obtaining specific qualifications was not requested, I ended up with a large amount of interesting data which were difficult to classify and code.

In addition, because I had not appreciated that the entry into nurse teaching was so varied (it seemed more complex than entry into midwifery teaching) this problem was compounded. The data obtained were subsequently found to be of little value to the study, and as such the analysis and findings have been omitted. A further pilot study in the initial stages may have highlighted that the question needed refining.

Degree studies

The question sought to establish whether respondents already held degrees, were in the process of studying for a degree, or intended to take up degree study within a two-year period. Overall, the findings for both cohorts were similar throughout and are reproduced in Tables 10.2–10.4.

An examination of the data reveals that 14 (47 per cent) of the midwife teacher, and 13 (43 per cent) of the nurse teacher cohorts already possessed a degree of some description. Of these, one midwife teacher and three nurse teachers had obtained degrees prior to entering the nursing profession while a further midwife teacher had undertaken degree studies combined

Table 10.2 Present and intended degree study of midwife/nurse teacher cohorts

	RMT cohort (30)		RNT cohort (30)		Both cohorts (60)	
	No.	*%*	*No.*	*%*	*No.*	*%*
Already possess a degree	14	47	13	43	27	45
Do not possess a degree but in the process of studying for one	11	37	8	26	19	32
Possess a degree and currently undertaking further degree study	7	23	2	7	9	15
Do not possess a degree but intend to start studying within the next two years	3	10	4	13	7	12
Possess a degree already, not currently studying, but intend to undertake further degree study within the next two years	6	20	4	13	10	17
Possess a degree already, not currently studying and not intending to undertake further degree study	1	3	7	23	8	13
Do not possess a degree and do not intend undertaking degree study	2	7	5	17	7	12

with nurse training. The remainder had all obtained degrees since completing nurse or midwifery training. The study did not seek to identify how many had acquired degrees prior to, or after, obtaining teacher status.

Eighteen (60 per cent) of the midwife teachers were currently undertaking degree study compared with 10 (33 per cent) of the nurse teachers. Of these 11 (37 per cent) midwife teachers and eight (26 per cent) nurse teachers were studying for an initial degree (Table 10.2). If those currently undertaking degree study successfully complete their degrees 77 per cent of the entire population will possess graduate status within the next three to four years.

Nine (30 per cent) midwife teachers and eight (27 per cent) nurse teachers not currently studying for a degree intended undertaking degree study within the following two years. This would entail initial degree study for three (10 per cent) of the midwife teachers and four (13 per cent) of the

Table 10.3　Classification of degrees

	RMT cohort (30)		RNT cohort (30)		Both cohorts (60)	
	No.	%	No.	%	No.	%
Already held						
Bachelors degree alone	8	27	7	23	15	25
Masters degree alone	3	10	3	10	6	10
Bachelors and Masters degree	3	10	2	7	5	8
Bachelors, Masters and PhD	0	0	1	3	1	2
Under current study						
No degree at present						
Studying for a Bachelors degree	2	7	4	13	6	10
Studying for a Masters degree	9	30	4	13	13	22
Undertaking higher degrees						
Possess a Bachelors degree and studying for a Masters degree	6	20	2	7	8	13
Possess a Bachelors and Masters degree, studying for a PhD	1	3	0	0	1	2

Table 10.4　Present degree study and future projections

	RMT cohort (30)		RNT cohort (30)		Both cohorts (60)	
	No.	%	No.	%	No.	%
Already possess a degree	14	47	13	43	27	45
Currently undertaking degree study (any level)	18	60	10	33	28	47
Not currently studying but intending to undertake degree study within the next two years	9	30	8	27	17	28
Total who will hold degree status if intentions to undertake study within the next two years are realized and completed successfully	28	93	25	83	53	88
Do not possess a degree and not intending to study in the future	2	7	5	17	7	12

nurse teachers. The remainder would be taking higher degrees. Again, if intentions are fully realized 53 (88 per cent) of the entire population should obtain degree status within the next five to six years.

Two (7 per cent) midwife teachers and five (17 per cent) nurse teachers did not possess a degree and did not intend studying for one. Both the midwifery participants and three of the nurse participants were over the age of 55 years. The remaining two nurse teachers were both over 45 years of age.

Classification of the type of degree under study is outlined in Table 10.3. It was interesting to note that 12 (40 per cent) of the midwife teachers and seven (23 per cent) of the nurse teachers either had, or anticipated, progressing directly to a higher degree. This is enlarged upon in the later discussion.

Motivation for undertaking degree study

Analysis of this question was more difficult than previous questions as something less tangible was being measured (Table 10.5). Responses did not necessarily require all boxes to be completed, therefore, simple proportioning was not appropriate. Those teachers who did not possess and did not intend to obtain a degree were asked not to complete this question.

Both groups had prioritized at least three items (some had prioritized 10)

Table 10.5   Motivation for undertaking degree study

If you hold a degree, or are studying for one at present, were your decisions to undertake further studies influenced by any of the following? (please tick those thought to be relevant and rank in order of priority):

	Tick	*Priority*
1. To broaden experience	☐	☐
2. To gain promotion	☐	☐
3. To improve personal image with colleagues	☐	☐
4. For personal growth	☐	☐
5. To socialize with other professionals	☐	☐
6. To provide stimulation not present in job	☐	☐
7. For the love of learning	☐	☐
8. U.K.C.C. recommendation (Project 2000)	☐	☐
9. To gain academic credibility	☐	☐
10. Other (please specify):	☐	☐

Additional Comments:

and from the total number of responses; the popularity of each item was determined (Table 10.6).

A weighted ranking analysis (Swinscow, 1980) of the first three priorities was carried out to confirm numerical ranking. It was also felt that this would give a more accurate picture of true motivating factors (Table 10.7).

For both the midwife and nurse teacher groups, using both methods of analysis, items 4, 1 and 7 were the main motivating factors (in that order). Rank order was subsequently slightly different for both groups.

Several of the cohort included 'other' in their choices clarifying their selection with the following reasons:

- interest in the subject;
- stimulation of discussion with non-nursing degree students;
- personal challenge/enjoyment;
- to occupy spare time;
- wanted to experience university education;
- understand the academic world.

It is generally accepted that when motivation for learning is intrinsic it is more likely to sustain students during further study than when it is extrinsic (Houle, 1961). Therefore, an attempt was made to ascertain whether learning for this population was intrinsically or extrinsically motivated.

When studying the characteristics of adults seeking additional learning, Houle classified them into the three categories: learner orientated, activity orientated and goal orientated. A comparison of the main motivating factors with the categories described by Houle confirms that the main characteristics for this population when seeking additional learning, fell into the learner orientated group (Table 10.8). The main motivating factors

Table 10.6 Total number of responses for each question

Question Number	1	2	3	4	5	6	7	8	9	10
Total responses from RMTs	22	3	1	27	6	3	10	4	1	7
Total responses from RNTs	15	2	0	25	0	3	12	8	11	1
Rank order RMTs	2	7	9	1	5	7	3	6	9	4
Rank order RNTs	2	7	9	1	9	6	3	5	4	8

Table 10.7 Priority ranking of first three responses

Question Number	1	2	3	4	5	6	7	8	9	10
Rank order RMTs	2	8	10	1	5	7	3	6	9	4
Rank order RNTs	2	6	9	1	9	7	3	5	4	8

Table 10.8 Original list reproduced with rank order of cohorts and Houle's categories added

	Rank RMTs	Order RNTs	Houle Cats
1. Broaden experience	2	2	LO
2. Gain promotion	8	6	GO
3. Improve personal image with colleagues	10	9	AO
4. Personal growth	1	1	LO
5. Socialize with other professionals	5	9	AO
6. Provide stimulation not present in job	7	7	AO
7. For the love of learning	3	3	LO
8. U.K.C.C. recommendation (Project 2000)	6	5	GO
9. To gain academic credibility	9	4	GO
10. Other (please specify)	4	8	Mixed

LO = Learner orientated; GO = Goal orientated; AO = Activity orientated

for this group appeared to be intrinsic, rather than extrinsic, and the hypothesis was disproved.

Support available for degree study

This question sought to establish how much study leave and financial support was available to those involved in degree study, during their professional careers. Those who undertook degree studies prior to coming into nursing have been omitted.

Results showed that sources of funding varied considerably between and within, both cohorts. Study leave was a much more stable entity. In percentaging out the responses to this question the picture emerges as in Table 10.9.

Although funding had been widely sought by both groups, a substantial proportion were unsuccessful and funded themselves entirely. Several participants commented that the battle to obtain funding was both time-consuming and demoralizing. Of the nurse teacher group 17 per cent did not request any funding as they wished to undertake degrees unrelated to nursing. Semi-structured interviews revealed that where financial support was received, this usually covered course costs and sometimes also included a book allowance and/or travelling expenses.

It was commendable that a high percentage of both groups had been granted study leave, although the amount of time was usually restricted to the length of study day and academic term time. Of the nurse teacher group 22 per cent commented that although study leave had been granted, its benefit was often eroded by heavy work loads.

When undertaking a second degree the midwife teacher group fared

Table 10.9 Support obtained for each degree

	Initial Degree		Second Degree		Third Degree	
	RMTs	RNTs	RMTs	RNTs	RMTs	RNTs
Financial support from employing authority	20	28	13	20	0	0
Financial support from a scholarship, etc.	20	11	50	0	100	100
Combination of above	4	17	12	40	0	0
No financial support at all	56	44	25	40	0	0
Study leave from employing authority	100	89	100	100	100	100

slightly better in funding than the nurse teacher group (75 per cent as opposed to 60 per cent). A surprising feature was that 50 per cent of the midwife teacher group, and none of the nurse teacher group, obtained funding from a scholarship. Possibly there are greater demands on scholarships available to nurses than there are for midwives. Conversely, it may just reflect the small numbers of those currently undertaking second degrees seen in this study (eight midwife teachers and five nurse teachers). All obtained study leave under the same conditions as those undertaking initial degree study.

The amount of support available for those undertaking a third degree showed an entirely different pattern, all receiving both funding and study leave. However, numbers were extremely small (two and one respectively) making it impossible to generalize.

Attitudes towards degree study

This section contains 18 items which seek to explore attitudes towards degree study. A Lickert type scale was used to quantify responses. Although not requested many additional comments were added by respondents which have been incorporated into the study.

Possession of a degree should be mandatory for all midwife and nurse teachers (Table 10.10)

The great majority of both midwife and nurse teachers agreed with this statment which was designed to correlate to the proposal in Project 2000. The nurse teacher cohort would appear to have firmer views in categorizing their choice from the very small percentage who were undecided.

Degree studies should be funded by the individual (Table 10.11)

A substantial number of both cohorts were undecided, or disagreed, that degree study should be funded by the individual. Nurse teacher responses were much more clear cut than those of midwife teachers. Several respondents commented that individuals should pay a proportionate amount towards degree study. This correlates fairly well to replies given for Table 10.15.

Degree studies should be funded by the employing authority (Table 10.12)

Responses for this statement were not as clear cut with a third of respondents being undecided and subsequently making it difficult to draw firm

Table 10.10

	RMTs (30)		RNTs (30)	
	No.	%	No.	%
Strongly agree	7	23	11	37
Agree	14	47	12	40
Undecided	5	17	1	3
Disagree	2	7	6	20
Strongly disagree	2	7	0	0

Table 10.11

	RMTs (30)		RNTs (30)	
	No.	%	No.	%
Strongly agree	2	7	1	3
Agree	7	23	2	7
Undecided	16	53	3	10
Disagree	5	17	18	60
Strongly disagree	0	0	6	20

Table 10.12

	RMTs (30)		RNTs (30)	
	No.	%	No.	%
Strongly agree	5	17	6	20
Agree	9	30	12	40
Undecided	11	36	10	33
Disagree	5	17	1	3
Strongly disagree	0	0	1	3

conclusions. Many of the respondents in both groups who fell into the agree category clarified their statements signifying that the employing authority should only pay if the degree were related to the sphere of work.

Degree studies should be funded by the English National Board (Table 10.13)

Two-thirds of both cohorts agreed with this statement while the remainder were undecided or disagreed. There was a surprising reversal of disagrees and undecided responses between each group indicating that midwife teachers felt more strongly than their nursing colleagues that the ENB should be responsible for degree funding. A number of respondents (30 and 40 per cent) added that this was an appropriate source of funding should degree status become mandatory, especially for first degrees.

Funding for degree studies should be negotiated by the individual from other available sources (e.g. scholarships, local authority, etc.) (Table 10.14)

It was difficult to draw firm conclusions from this question because of the spread of responses. The nurse teacher cohort were much more definite in strongly disagreeing. This may account for the smaller number applying for scholarships in the previous section.

The last three items might have generated more valid information if

Table 10.13

	RMTs (30)		RNTs (30)	
	No.	%	No.	%
Strongly agree	3	10	4	13
Agree	15	50	14	47
Undecided	10	33	1	3
Disagree	1	3	10	33
Strongly disagree	1	3	1	3

Table 10.14

	RMTs (30)		RNTs (30)	
	No.	%	No.	%
Strongly agree	3	10	2	7
Agree	13	43	13	43
Undecided	5	17	3	10
Disagree	8	27	5	17
Strongly disagree	1	3	7	23

respondents had been asked to prioritize the most appropriate source of funding from a specified list. Semi-structured interviews indicated that funding should be a shared responsibility between the individual, the employer and the ENB. Obtaining funding from other sources was experienced as being 'time-consuming', 'demoralizing' and leaving a feeling of 'rejection' if not successful (participants' comments).

If only a proportion of funding were available, what proportion would be a reasonable amount for the individual to pay? (Table 10.15)

A high percentage of both cohorts indicated that between 25 and 50 per cent of funding would be a reasonable proportion for the individual to contribute towards degree study. This correlates well with the attitudes expressed earlier that funding should be a shared responsibility between the individual and the employer, especially if degree status should become mandatory for teaching staff.

As professionals, midwife and nurse teachers should strive for degree status regardless of funding from outside sources (Table 10.16)

A larger proportion of both cohorts agreed with this statement although the margins between those disagreeing, or undecided, were not as clear cut as

Table 10.15

| | RMTs (30) | | RNTs (30) | |
	No.	%	No.	%
None	0	0	1	3
Approximately 25%	15	50	4	13
Approximately 50%	11	37	19	63
Approximately 75%	2	7	1	3
Approximately 100%	2	7	4	13
Other	0	0	1	3

Table 10.16

| | RMTs (30) | | RNTs (30) | |
	No.	%	No.	%
Strongly agree	6	20	4	13
Agree	13	43	12	40
Undecided	5	17	5	17
Disagree	5	17	8	27
Strongly disagree	1	3	1	3

anticipated. The author had expected this question to correlate more closely with the responses given for Table 10.11. However, this was not the case. Possibly the question would have benefited from more refinement with different wording.

Time off for degree studies should be provided for by the employer (Table 10.17)

This statement achieved a strongly positive reply from both cohorts. The midwife teacher who was undecided added the comment that time off should only be given if the degree were related to health care. Of those who disagreed none was contemplating degree study. One made the comment: 'why should colleagues carry those doing degrees', and another: 'not if the degree is un-related to the job'.

Individuals should be prepared to spend a large proportion of their own time studying for a degree (Table 10.18)

Midwife teacher responses were much less well cut than nurse teachers. A surprisingly large number of midwife teachers (37 per cent) disagreed with the statement, leading the author to wonder if the statement was ambiguous. Interviews revealed that a proportion had taken it to mean no study leave support from the employing authority. This introduced a measure of

Table 10.17

	RMTs (30)		RNTs (30)	
	No.	%	No.	%
Strongly agree	17	57	19	63
Agree	12	40	9	30
Undecided	1	3	0	0
Disagree	0	0	1	3
Strongly disagree	0	0	1	3

Table 10.18

	RMTs (30)		RNTs (30)	
	No.	%	No.	%
Strongly agree	0	0	4	13
Agree	12	40	14	47
Undecided	7	23	4	13
Disagree	9	30	5	17
Strongly disagree	2	7	3	10

unreliability into the results as not all of the cohort was interviewed. Overall the nurse teacher group possibly have a more practical outlook!

Information about degress should be provided by the employer
(Table 10.19)

Although the spread of responses for this statement was fairly even, approximately half of both cohorts either did not agree or were undecided. Comments included that it should be a part of career advice and professional development, while some felt people should be sufficiently motivated to discover what was available for themselves. The earlier literature review has indicated that the uptake of further education is greater when career advice is given, therefore the negative response rates were surprising.

The degree being studied for should be related to some aspect of midwifery or nursing (Table 10.20)

Midwife teacher responses were evenly split between agreeing and disagreeing with this statement with only a small proportion being undecided. A larger percentage of their nursing counterparts either agreed with the statement or were undecided. One respondent commented that the statement presented a narrow view and that any degree would do. Other

Table 10.19

| | RMTs (30) | | RNTs (30) | |
	No.	%	No.	%
Strongly agree	6	20	4	13
agree	7	23	12	40
Undecided	7	23	6	20
Disagree	8	27	7	23
Strongly disagree	2	7	1	3

Table 10.20

| | RMTs (30) | | RNTs (30) | |
	No.	%	No.	%
Strongly agree	5	17	6	20
Agree	9	30	10	33
Undecided	2	7	5	17
Disagree	12	40	6	20
Strongly disagree	2	7	3	10

comments indicated that people would do better if they were studying an area of particular interest to them or that if funding was provided by the ENB or the employing authority the degree should be related to some aspect of health care.

Individuals should undertake whichever degree they are interested in (Table 10.21)

Overall, both groups responded positively to this statement. This appeared to be somewhat at variance with the response to the previous question. It may have been better if respondents were asked to specify either/or for these two items as they contain opposing statements. This was corroborated, to an extent, during interviews. Comments indicated that if support was given by the ENB or the employer, then the choice of degree should be negotiated to meet the needs of both the individual and the organization.

The possession of a degree is necessary to maintain professional credibility (Table 10.22)

Again, responses from both cohorts were positive rather than negative. Attitudes would appear to approximate, to an extent, to the current degree study trends seen in the previous section.

Table 10.21

	RMTs (30)		RNTs (30)	
	No.	%	No.	%
Strongly agree	7	23	5	17
Agree	14	47	13	43
Undecided	2	7	4	13
Disagree	7	23	4	13
Strongly disagree	0	0	4	13

Table 10.22

	RMTs (30)		RNTs (30)	
	No.	%	No.	%
Strongly agree	6	20	8	27
Agree	14	47	10	33
Undecided	3	10	7	23
Disagree	6	20	5	17
Strongly disagree	1	3	0	0

Possession of a degree should be reflected by an appropriate increase in salary (Table 10.23)

A substantial number of both cohorts were in agreement with this statement. Nurse teachers were, once again, more definite in their views than their midwife counterparts. A proportion of those agreeing qualified their response by stating that this should only occur if the degree were related to the profession or if it improved performance. Two respondents felt that having a degree did not necessarily effectively contribute anything of worth to the organization, therefore, should not warrant extra salary.

Individuals studying for a degree should share their knowledge with their peers (Table 10.24)

A high measure of agreement was obtained across both groups on this statement. No respondents disagreed but 3 per cent of the midwife teacher group and 7 per cent of hte nurse teacher group were undecided. The responses would indicate a committed willingness to share knowledge with colleagues, thus enhancing learning. One respondent felt that this question could infringe on the rights of the individual.

Table 10.23

| | RMTs (30) | | RNTs (30) | |
	No.	%	No.	%
Strongly agree	3	10	8	27
Agree	17	57	13	43
Undecided	6	20	1	3
Disagree	4	13	6	20
Strongly disagree	0	0	2	7

Table 10.24

| | RMTs (30) | | RNTs (30) | |
	No.	%	No.	%
Strongly agree	17	57	16	53
Agree	12	40	12	40
Undecided	1	3	2	7
Disagree	0	0	0	0
Strongly disagree	0	0	0	0

What is learnt when undertaking a degree is the 'private property' of the individual (Table 10.25)

It was commendable that this statement achieved a high measure of disagreement among both cohorts. The one respondent who agreed with the statement clarified the response by stating that if the individual had received no support at all the degree should be classified as 'private property'. Responses correlated very well with the previous item.

What is learnt when undertaking a degree should be used to enhance midwifery and nursing education (Table 10.26)

A high measure of agreement was again evident, giving further credence to the beliefs expressed in Tables 10.24 and 10.25. It also emphasized the overall impression that colleagues were very willing to share their knowledge with their peers and with those undergoing the learning process. Of those who disagreed, several comments were added relating this to how funding was administered.

Undertaking degree studies widens the individual's range of job opportunities (Table 10.27)

Once again answers were clear cut in each cohort with a substantial measure of agreement being achieved. A number of the nurse teacher cohort

Table 10.25

| | RMTs (30) | | RNTs (30) | |
	No.	%	No.	%
Strongly agree	0	0	0	0
Agree	0	0	1	3
Undecided	3	10	2	7
Disagree	17	57	12	40
Strongly disagree	10	33	15	50

Table 10.26

| | RMTs (30) | | RNTs (30) | |
	No.	%	No.	%
Strongly agree	15	50	13	43
Agree	14	47	16	53
Undecided	1	3	1	3
Disagree	0	0	0	0
Strongly disagree	0	0	0	0

Table 10.27

| | RMTs (30) | | RNTs (30) | |
	No.	*%*	*No.*	*%*
Strongly agree	6	20	9	30
Agree	22	73	16	53
Undecided	2	7	5	17
Disagree	0	0	0	0
Strongly disagree	0	0	0	0

who were undecided said this depended on the degree gained, the job applied for and the individual's circumstances. The correlation to the numbers in both cohorts of those presently undertaking degree study is clear.

Discussion, conclusions and recommendations

The major finding of this research was that the motivating factors behind degree study for both the nurse and midwife teacher cohorts were intrinsic, rather than extrinsic. Data analysis revealed that the most popular reasons for undertaking further study of this nature were to foster personal growth, to broaden experience and for the love of learning. The hypothesis was, therefore, disproved.

The research indicates quite clearly that teachers in this study group were being pro-active in their efforts to obtain degrees, rather than driven by the thought (threat) of legislation. Although possible legislation was taken into account it appeared to be only a minor consideration. These findings related well to other studies on motivation, which generally found that health professionals were more likely to continue their education beyond initial training to improve their practice, rather than because of imposed legislation.

For this population, adult characteristics for seeking higher education were mainly learner orientated, thus more likely to sustain the population in their efforts to obtain academic excellence. This would suggest that should the proposed mandatory graduate status for nurse teaching become a reality, there would not be too much opposition from those working in this field. The legislative process would only be required to stimulate the small percentage of teachers less likely to undertake this route.

Buttigieg (1990) estimated that 80.5 per cent of senior nurse educators agree that nurse teaching should be a graduate profession. The attitude survey revealed that 70.5 per cent of nurse and midwife teachers (across a variety of grades) held similar views, and concurred that degree status should be mandatory for nurse educators.

Peters (1977) suggests that degree study instils an attitude towards learning which gives the individual wider educational opportunity in the future. The percentage of respondents in this study who either had, were in the process of, or intended to build on earlier degree study, would give some credence to this belief. A large percentage of the population studied also believed that possession of a degree widened the individual's job opportunities. A review of job advertisements for senior posts in nursing (teaching and service) also indicates that degree possession is becoming increasingly important if one wishes to progress up the career ladder to the higher echelons.

Degree study is designed to advance knowledge and understanding, to stimulate intellectual thought, encourage critical awareness, foster empirical study and give an all-round depth of knowledge to those involved (Peters, 1977). The UKCC Code of Professional Conduct (UKCC, 1984) reminds nurses that they are individually accountable for their professional development. This also extends to those in nurse education who have a dual professional responsibility both as nurses and teachers.

Nursing has, for many years, been identified by its vocational and practical image. However, in the last two to three decades nurses have consistently endeavoured to raise their image by achieving professional status (Chapman, 1977; Pyne, 1981). It would seem that there is a similar dichotomy for those concerned with professional education.

Jarvis (1983, p. 22) offers his own definition of a professional as 'one who continually seeks the mastery of a branch of learning upon which his occupation is based, so that he may offer a service to his client'. Implicit in this definition is the belief that one of the hallmarks of professionalism is an attempt at excellence achieved through further (continuing) education. The trends inherent in this research show that nurse and midwife educators are already well on the way to achieving graduate status and developing an all-degree teaching profession in nursing.

Buttigieg (1990) reports that 29.5 per cent of her student teacher cohort already possessed a degree with a further 3.9 per cent in the process of obtaining graduate status. Of her cohort 70 per cent intended studying for a first or higher degree on completion of their teacher training course. Kershaw (1990a) quotes a figure of 50 per cent for current qualified teachers already possessing a degree while my own research has shown that 45 per cent of the entire cohort already had a degree but that this figure would increase to 76.5 per cent within the next two to three years. A further 12 per cent of my cohort of teachers would commence studying for degrees within this time span, leaving only 11.5 per cent of the teacher population without degree status. None of these was in the lower age groups and would naturally be phased out through retirement.

Trends in degree study patterns between student teachers in the study undertaken by Buttigieg (1990) and qualified teachers in this study are relatively compatible and highlight that teaching staff in nursing have been continuing their professional development of their own volition.

Equal proportions of nurse and midwife teachers already held degree status (43 and 47 per cent), but 10 per cent of both groups had opted to bypass a first degree and progress directly to higher degree status. A considerably larger proportion of midwife teachers were currently studying for degrees (60 per cent) than the nurse teacher group (33 per cent) and within these cohorts a large percentage were opting not to undertake first degrees (50 per cent of midwife teachers and 40 per cent of nurse teachers currently studying). This may not be the wisest course of action to take, as a first degree is generally thought to give the basic all-round academic grounding required for higher degree study (Kershaw, 1990b).

Just under 50 per cent of both cohorts agreed that information about degree study should be provided by the employer. This was a surprising response but, in retrospect, the question was not worded in such a way as to give me the information being sought. If it had been related more concisely to career advice and professional development, ultimate responses might have been different. With the large numbers of teachers in the study going directly for higher degrees, perhaps educational managers should re-think any advice they wish to offer potential teachers, or qualified teachers working within their institutions. Similarly, perhaps the UKCC should be more specific in what they mean by an all-graduate teaching profession.

The tendency to bypass a first degree may be related both to the length of degree courses and financial considerations. However, this finding was not anticipated and the questionnaire was not designed to examine this issue. Certainly, funding was found to be unequally and haphazardly administered. Interviews revealed that many thought this was on a 'first come, first served' basis rather than any attempt being made to look at individual, professional needs or the needs of the organization. The attitude survey highlighted that a large proportion of both cohorts did not feel that individuals should fund their own degree studies, especially if this became mandatory requirement. However, both cohorts were quite willing for this to be a shared commitment between the individual and (preferably) the ENB.

Possibly the ENB should consider stipulating that teacher preparation courses should be incorporated into degree courses of a modular nature where, if appropriate, credits such as those given by the Council for National Academic Awards (CNAA, 1990) can be given for prior learning. The ENB and employing authorities could also take on board the earlier comments relating to obtaining funding fom outside sources as this type of activity could be a de-motivating factor for those wishing to undertake academic study.

It was interesting that although 73 per cent of the sample agreed that degree status should be a mandatory requirement for nurse educators, only

58 per cent felt that, as professionals, they should strive for degree status regardless of funding from other sources. This is possibly related to financial constraints and the mere practicality of not being in debt as a consequence of undertaking higher education.

Study leave was a more stable entity than funding and the employing authorities must be commended for their willingness to make this provision. Both cohorts were strongly in favour of receiving study leave and this is probably a more important consideration than receiving funding. The high percentage of teachers undertaking degrees possibly cushions the extra work load involved, on a simple reciprocative basis, in covering for colleagues when on study days. However, as the move is towards a more student-centred educational approach (ENB, 1989), consideration should be given by employing authorities to the increased amount of teaching time that this takes. Possibly some short-term funding should be provided to allow extra teachers to be employed while others are obtaining degree status.

Erosion of study leave time due to pressure of work was more evident among the nurse teacher that the midwife teacher group and may deserve special consideration. On the other hand, to be practical, news reports of the current financial state of the National Health Service do not indicate that this will be a top priority, but it should not be forgotten. Perhaps nurse and midwife educators are becoming more profesional in seeing this as part of their own professional development, for which they have the main responsibility. However, the study indicates that if degree status is to become mandatory and financial help is not available then an appropriate increase in salary should be given to recompense individuals for the expenses incurred.

The research showed that the motivating factors for nurse and midwife teachers to obtain degree status were similar and being achieved by a large proportion. The UKCC (1987) does not specify that the degree studied should be related to nursing (it does not necessarily need to be in teaching) and this research indicates mixed views on the topic. Some felt quite strongly that if time off and funding were provided, then the degree should be allied to health care. It is reasonable to expect that the organization should gain some benefit if funding for degree study is provided by them or the ENB. Academic attainment and motivation, however, may be just as valuable if a wide range of degrees is obtained, and may allow nurses and midwives to function more comfortably in the higher education sector. This issue is not addressed in the UKCC (1987) proposals.

Senior nurse educators should start considering what level of degree is appropriate for their teaching staff and should incorporate suitable advice into the performance review. Some guidelines from the UKCC would also be of benefit. I would suggest that although the possession of degrees is likely to enhance professional credibility, careful consideration should be given to how teachers are supported while they achieve this objective and a large, longitudinal, study should be undertaken to establish the true benefits of an all-degree teaching profession once degree status is mandatory.

Critique/limitations of the study

This research has provided an interesting 'snap-shot' of the trends in degree study for nurse and midwife teachers. The survey approach proved an appropriate research method to use as the issues explored involved systematic observation of the research population in a natural environment. The intention was to obtain information which could be analysed and from which patterns could be extracted and comparisons made. In describing the characteristics of a randomly selected population of nurse and midwife teachers, it was anticipated that some relationships and answers (on degree study) would emerge which were common to the group as a whole. The information to be gained was of a personal, tangible nature and, as such, was unsuitable for experimental research.

Techniques for data gathering did allow a large amount of information to be collected within a relatively short period of time, at minimal cost. The use of pre-coded questionnaires ensured anonymity while confidentiality was assured when questionnaires were posted. This approach was felt to be advantageous as it encouraged participants to provide honest answers. Some of the comments proferred certainly gave the impression that respondents did not feel in any way constrained!

The questionnaire did not always generate the data required, so that some results were rendered meaningless and served only to generate unnecessary work. A question had been included to elicit what professional and teaching qualifications the sample population held. This was to serve primarily as a check that everyone met the teaching criteria for inclusion into the study. I also wanted to see if any significant patterns of further study emerged or if there was an overall picture evolving of the routes taken in order to qualify as a teacher. Basic nursing and midwifery qualifications were easy to code and analyse but diploma study and teaching qualifications were considerably more complicated and difficult to analyse.

It has been noted earlier in this chapter that it is not always possible to examine all the variables within a situation and that the wrong choice can complicate, or even invalidate the research. This occurred in the present study where particular problems arose, as outlined above, with the statistical data analysis on the question of professional qualifications. Insufficient attention had been paid to the number of existing variables within the question and too much inappropriate information was generated. In consequence, some of the data could not be classified and used in the study. Fortunately, this did not affect the outcome of the research, but one has to ask whether the inclusion of this question was really relevant. However, it does highlight the importance of defining the purpose of the study and the careful preparation needed in questionnaire design.

All questions on the questionnaire were designed to allow respondents to complete them quickly while at the same time generating the information I wanted. However, the particular question mentioned above (Figure 10.1) did not take account of the changes in legislation over the life span of the teachers concerned, or the combination of ways that nurses can now qualify to become teachers.

This is embarrassingly exemplified by the fact that raw data, collated to estimate the number of Registered Nurse Teachers (RNTs) in the study, revealed more RNTs than the study population. This could have been because midwife teachers also held an RNT qualification but this was not

---

Professional and Teaching Qualifications

PLEASE CIRCLE ALL WHICH APPLY

1. SRN/RGN

2. SCM/RM

3. RMN

4. RSCN

5. Health Visitors Certificate

6. Joint Board of Clinical Nursing Studies Courses (please specify) _____

    _____

7. English National Board Courses (please specify) _____

    _____

    _____

8. Professional Diplomas (please specify) _____

    _____

9. Registered Nurse Teacher (RNT)

10. Registered Midwife Teacher (RMT)

11. Certificate of Education (please specify) _____

    _____

12. Post Graduate Certificate in the Education of Adults

    Other (please specify) _____

    _____

Figure 10.1

the case. In order to overcome this problem in future it may be necessary to ensure that the possible responses are mutually exclusive. Possibly another way would have been to ask respondents to give dates of qualification, or to ask them to list their routes into nurse education.

If I were to undertake a similar, subsequent study, I would ensure that I had examined in greater detail exactly what data I wished to generate along with their relevance to the outcome of the study. Although the information collected (for this particular question) was interesting, and indicated that nurse teachers were very committed to extending their own continuing education, it did not really tell me anything about what motivates teachers to undertake degree study. Therefore, I must conclude that the bulk of the collected information was irrelevant.

Certain questions yielded unexpected results and may have been better if the wording had been more specific. These have been discussed, where they occur, in the findings. It is acknowledged that further piloting of the questionnaire may have eliminated some of these discrepancies.

The use of interviews proved to be of value in that it enabled the researcher to explore, in greater depth, some of the issues raised on the questionnaire. This technique is nevertheless quite time-consuming to undertake and the recording of data is sometimes tedious. Only a small proportion of the sample population was interviewed and it is recognized that, although randomly selected, they may not be indicative of the group as a whole.

In retrospect I wish that more time had been available both to spend on refining the research tools and to enable a larger population to be surveyed. This may have generated results with greater validity and upon which wider general recommendations could be made. I suspect that I was too ambitious from the start and it might have been advantageous to have delayed the study until I was less constrained by the stresses of completing a substantial project, for assessment purposes, in a short period of time.

I had the advantage of having conducted a similar, smaller study the year previously but, as stated, had not fully appreciated the inherent differences between nurse and midwife teachers, or their routes of entry into this field. I would like to advise others having to undertake such a piece of research to think carefully about the time span available for completing their project. It is essential to draw up, and adhere to, a written action plan, to clarify at an early stage exactly what new information they are trying to generate and to read widely around their chosen research subject area. Also they need to ensure that they have adequate on-going supervision from someone well versed in the intricacies of research work, who can advise on both the feasibility of the work to be undertaken and the suitability of the chosen research method.

I would also advise others not to be reticent in seeking answers to questions from a variety of expert sources (professionals, managers, statisticians, librarians, etc.) and to ensure that some back-up support (family, colleagues, friends, etc.) is available. Embarking on research should not be undertaken lightly, or by the faint-hearted, as the best results are usually generated by those who are committed to what they are doing. However, for anyone wishing to advance knowledge, the whole research process can be very worthwhile. Although I have not carried out many research projects, personal experience has proved that it can be most enjoyable and an excellent way to extend one's own learning.

The use of the survey method in this research did generate valid answers to the questions posed at the beginning of the study. The research indicates that the causal relationship for nurse and midwife teachers undertaking degree study was intrinsic and learner orientated. It would be interesting to carry out a further study on a much wider nurse/midwife teacher population to see if the findings could be replicated and substantiated.

I went through many anxious phases while undertaking the original work, ranging from worries that the topic was inappropriate, anxiety over lack of practical experience in carrying out research and fear that insufficient numbers would complete the questionnaires. This was compounded by constraints on the amount of time available to undertake the work and the knowledge that on 'judgement day' success, or failure, would probably affect the standard of degree awarded. However, despite all of this, I enjoyed carrying out the project (some fears were unfounded) and learnt a great deal more about the practicalities of research and the problems that can be encountered along the line.

I must say that I was very relieved when the research was finally completed and was also pleased with the end results. Printing out the final thesis took much longer than I had anticipated, as did proof-reading the text . . . something else for others to keep in mind if they are constrained by time. I was often sustained and encouraged by family, friends and colleagues and valued their support and the interest shown in the work undertaken. Similar support was also given by appropriate experts in research and statistics which was both invaluable and accepted gratefully.

Writing this chapter has allowed me to look more critically at the original aims of the work and has proved an even greater learning experience. It has certainly provided me with a great impetus to undertake further research and I would certainly wish to extend this encouragement to anyone embarking on research, either as a complete novice, or with little previous experience. Although not easy, the work involved can be both enjoyable and challenging, while also serving to increase and extend personal and scientific knowledge.

References

Abdellah F G and Levine E (1979) *Better Patient Care Through Nursing Research*, 2nd edn. Macmillan, New York.

Allan P (1987) The evolving curriculum in nursing education. In Allan P and Jolley M (Eds) *The Curriculum in Nursing Education*. Croom Helm, London, pp. 209–18.

Altschul A (1982) How far should further education go? *Nursing Mirror* 155 (1), 29–30.

Bell J (1987) *Doing Your Research Project*. Open University Press, Milton Keynes.

Best J W (1981) *Research in Education*, 4th edn. Prentice-Hall, Englewood Cliffs, NJ.

Brown L A (1988) Maintaining professional practice – is continuing education the cure or merely a tonic? *Nurse Education Today* 8 (5), 251–7.

Buttigieg M A (1990) *Teacher Preparation: An Evaluation of the Preparation of Teachers within Nursing, Midwifery and Health Visiting. A Report of a Survey and Evaluation*. English National Board, London.

Carlisle D (1991) Prepare for PREPP, 4: take five. *Nursing Times* 87 (6), 40–1.

Chapman C M (1977) Concepts of professionalism. *Journal of Advanced Nursing* 2 (1), 51–5.

Chiarella M (1990) Developing the credibility of continuing education. *Nurse Education Today* 10 (1), 70–3.

Cohen L and Manion L (1989) *Research Methods in Education*, 3rd edn. Routledge, London.

Commission on Nursing Education (1985) *The Education of Nurses: A New Dispensation*. RCN, London (Chairman, H. Judge).

Council for National Academic Awards (1990) *Handbook: 1990–1991*. CNAA, London.

Davidson L (1991) Prepare for PREPP. *Nursing Times* 87 (3), 50–2.

de Haven, M M (1990) Compliance with mandatory continuing edcuation in nursing: a hospital based study. *Journal of Continuing Education in Nursing* 21 (3), 102–4.

Department of Health (1989a) *Working for Patients*. HMSO, London (CM 555).

Department of Health (1989b) *Education and Training: Working Paper 10*. HMSO, London.

English National Board for Nursing, Midwifery and Health Visiting (1988) *Preparation of Teachers – Information Package*. (Circular 1988/63/MAT.). ENB, London.

English National Board for Nursing, Midwifery and Health Visiting (1989) *Project 2000 – 'A New Preparation for Practice'. Guidelines and Criteria for Course Development and the Formation of Collaborative Links Between Approved Training Institutions within the National Health Service and Centres of Higher Education*. ENB, London.

Faulkenberry J (1986) Marketing strategies to increase participation in continuing education. *Journal of Nursing Staff Development* 2 (3), 98–104.

Fox D J (1976) *Fundamentals of Research in Nursing*, 3rd edn. Appleton-Century-Croft, Norwalk, CT.

Friend B (1991) Prepare for PREPP 6: view from the top. *Nursing Times* 87 (8), 24–5.

Glaser B G and Strauss A L (1967) *The Discovery of Grounded Theory*. Aldine de Gruyter, New York.

Houle C O (1961) *The Inquiring Mind*. University of Wisconsin Press, Madison, WI.

Jarvis P (1983) *Professional Education*. Croom Helm, London.

Kershaw B (1990a) Project 2000 – what do trained staff need for its successful implementation and development? *Senior Nurse* 10 (1), 4–6.

Kershaw B (1990b) Degree level studies. In Kershaw, B. (Ed.) *Nursing Competence: A Guide to Professional Development*. Edward Arnold, London.

Lahiff M (1983) *Attitudes to the need for continuing education: paper presented at the*

RCN Association of Nursing Education Conference. Royal College of Nursing, London.

Lancaster A (1975) *Guidelines to Research in Nursing: No. 2 – An Introduction to the Research Process.* King Edward's Hostpial Fund, London.

Lathlean J and Farnish S (1984) *The Ward Sister Training Project: An Evaluation of a Training Scheme for Ward Sisters.* NERU Report No. 3. Nursing Education Research Unit, Chelsea College, London.

Mackereth P (1989) An investigation of the developmental influences on nurses' motivation for their continuing education. *Journal of Advanced Nursing* 14 (19), 776–87.

McCrea H (1989) Motivation for continuing education in midwifery. *Midwifery* 5 (3), 134–45.

McNeill P (1985) *Research Methods.* Tavistock, London.

Millonig V L (1985) Motivational orientation toward learning after graduation. *Nursing Administration Quarterly* 9 (4), 79–86.

Nie N H, Hull C H, Jenkinson J G, Steinbrenner K and Bent D H (1975) *Statistical Package for the Social Sciences.* McGraw-Hill, New York.

Nugent A B (1990) The need for continuing professional education for nurses. *Journal of Advanced Nursing* 15 (4), 471–7.

O'Connor A B (1979) Reasons nurses participate in continuing education. *Nursing Research* 28 (6), 354–9.

Oppenheim A N (1966) *Questionnaire Design and Attitude Measurement.* Heinemann, London.

Peters R S (1977) *Education and the Education of Teachers.* Routledge and Kegan Paul, London.

Popiel E S (1969) The many facets of continuing education in nursing. *Journal of Nursing Education* 8 (1), 3–13.

Pyne R H (1981) *Professional Discipline in Nursing.* Blackwell Scientific Publications, Oxford.

Reid N G and Boore J R P (1987) *Research Methods and Statistics in Health Care.* Edward Arnold, London.

Rogers J (1987) Limited opportunities. *Nursing Times* 83 (36), 31–2.

Rogers J and Lawrence J (1986) *Continuing Professional Education for Qualified Nurses, Midwives and Health Visitors: A Report of a Survey and Case Study.* Ashdale Press/ Austin Cornish, Peterborough.

Royal College of Nursing (1985) *Commission on nursing education. The education of nurses, a new dispensation* (Judge Report). RCN, London.

Smith V A (1990) An exploration of the factors which determine midwife teachers' reasons for pursuing degree qualifications. Unpublished Study.

Studdy S and Hunt C (1980) A computerised survey of learning needs. *Nursing Times* 76 (25), 1084–7.

Sweeney J F (1986) Nurse education: learner centred or teacher centred? *Nurse Education Today* 6 (6) 257–62.

Swinscow T D V (1980) *Statistics at Square One*, 6th edn. British Medical Association, London.

United Kingdom Central Council for Nursing, Midwifery and Health Visiting (1984) *Code of Professional Conduct for the Nurse, Midwife and Health Visitor*, 2nd edn. London, UKCC.

United Kingdom Central Council for Nursing, Midwifery and Health Visiting (1986) *Project 2000: A New Preparation for Practice.* UKCC, London.

United Kingdom Central Council for Nursing, Midwifery and Health Visiting (1987) *Project 2000: The Final Proposals. Project paper 9.* UKCC, London.

United Kingdom Central Council for Nursing, Midwifery and Health Visiting (1988) *Criteria and Associated Guidelines for the Recording of Qualifications for Nurse Tutor, Midwife Teacher, Lecturer in Health Visiting, District Nurse Tutor and Occupational Health Nurse Teacher.* (Circular PS&D/88/03). UKCC, London.

United Kingdom Central Council for Nursing, Midwifery and Health Visiting (1990) *The Report of the Post-registration Education and Practice Project.* UKCC, London.

Urbano M T (1988) What really motivates nurses to participate in mandatory professional continuing education? *Journal of Continuing Education in Nursing* 19 (1), 38–42.

Ward R (1990) Influencing attitudes among nurses taking higher education. *Senior Nurse* 10 (3), 24–5, 27.

Webster R (1990) The role of the nurse teacher. *Senior Nurse* 10 (8), 16–18.

Wilson K J W (1975) *Guidelines to Research in Nursing: No. 4 – An Introduction to Sampling and Statistical Concepts.* King Edward's Hospital Fund, London.

Index